S0-EID-104

PROTECTING OUR FORCES

Improving Vaccine Acquisition and Availability in the U.S. Military

Stanley M. Lemon, Susan Thaul, Salem Fisseha, and Heather C. O'Maonaigh, *Editors*

Committee on a Strategy for Minimizing the Impact of Naturally Occurring Infectious Diseases of Military Importance: Vaccine Issues in the U.S. Military

Medical Follow-up Agency

INSTITUTE OF MEDICINE
OF THE NATIONAL ACADEMIES

THE NATIONAL ACADEMIES PRESS
Washington, D.C.
www.nap.edu

THE NATIONAL ACADEMIES PRESS • 500 Fifth Street, N.W. • Washington, DC 20001

NOTICE: The project that is the subject of this report was approved by the Governing Board of the National Research Council, whose members are drawn from the councils of the National Academy of Sciences, the National Academy of Engineering, and the Institute of Medicine. The members of the committee responsible for the report were chosen for their special competences and with regard for appropriate balance.

Support for this project was provided by U.S. Army Medical Research and Materiel Command (Contract No. DAMD17-00-C-0003). The views presented in this report are those of the Institute of Medicine Committee on a Strategy for Minimizing the Impact of Naturally Occurring Infectious Diseases of Military Importance: Vaccine Issues in the U.S. Military and are not necessarily those of the funding agency.

International Standard Book Number 0-309-08499-7

Library of Congress Conrol Number 2002110509

Additional copies of this report are available for sale from the National Academies Press, 500 Fifth Street, N.W., Box 285, Washington, DC 20055. Call (800) 624-6242 or (202) 334-3313 (in the Washington metropolitan area); Internet: http://www.nap.edu.

For more information about the Institute of Medicine, visit the IOM home page at **www.iom.edu.**

Copyright 2002 by the National Academy of Sciences. All rights reserved.

Printed in the United States of America

The serpent has been a symbol of long life, healing, and knowledge among almost all cultures and religions since the beginning of recorded history. The serpent adopted as a logotype by the Institute of Medicine is a relief carving from ancient Greece, now held by the Staatliche Museen in Berlin.

"Knowing is not enough; we must apply.
Willing is not enough; we must do."

—Goethe

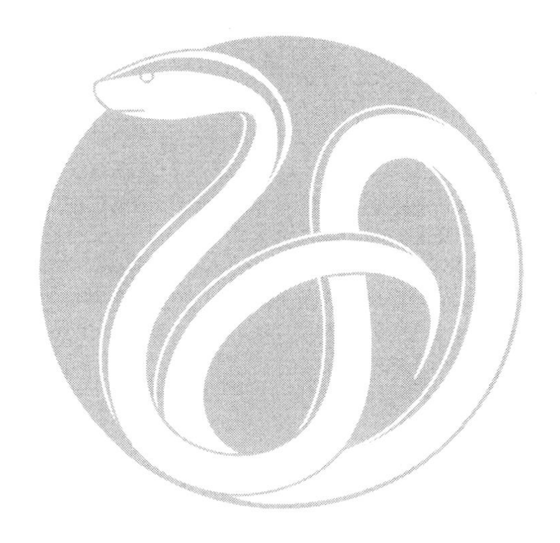

INSTITUTE OF MEDICINE
OF THE NATIONAL ACADEMIES

Shaping the Future for Health

THE NATIONAL ACADEMIES

Advisers to the Nation on Science, Engineering, and Medicine

The **National Academy of Sciences** is a private, nonprofit, self-perpetuating society of distinguished scholars engaged in scientific and engineering research, dedicated to the furtherance of science and technology and to their use for the general welfare. Upon the authority of the charter granted to it by the Congress in 1863, the Academy has a mandate that requires it to advise the federal government on scientific and technical matters. Dr. Bruce M. Alberts is president of the National Academy of Sciences.

The **National Academy of Engineering** was established in 1964, under the charter of the National Academy of Sciences, as a parallel organization of outstanding engineers. It is autonomous in its administration and in the selection of its members, sharing with the National Academy of Sciences the responsibility for advising the federal government. The National Academy of Engineering also sponsors engineering programs aimed at meeting national needs, encourages education and research, and recognizes the superior achievements of engineers. Dr. Wm. A. Wulf is president of the National Academy of Engineering.

The **Institute of Medicine** was established in 1970 by the National Academy of Sciences to secure the services of eminent members of appropriate professions in the examination of policy matters pertaining to the health of the public. The Institute acts under the responsibility given to the National Academy of Sciences by its congressional charter to be an adviser to the federal government and, upon its own initiative, to identify issues of medical care, research, and education. Dr. Harvey V. Fineberg is president of the Institute of Medicine.

The **National Research Council** was organized by the National Academy of Sciences in 1916 to associate the broad community of science and technology with the Academy's purposes of furthering knowledge and advising the federal government. Functioning in accordance with general policies determined by the Academy, the Council has become the principal operating agency of both the National Academy of Sciences and the National Academy of Engineering in providing services to the government, the public, and the scientific and engineering communities. The Council is administered jointly by both Academies and the Institute of Medicine. Dr. Bruce M. Alberts and Dr. Wm. A. Wulf are chair and vice chair, respectively, of the National Research Council.

www.national-academies.org

COMMITTEE ON A STRATEGY FOR MINIMIZING THE IMPACT OF NATURALLY OCCURRING INFECTIOUS DISEASES OF MILITARY IMPORTANCE: VACCINE ISSUES IN THE U.S. MILITARY

STANLEY M. LEMON, M.D. (*Chair*), Dean of Medicine and Professor, University of Texas Medical Branch, Galveston
CHARLES C. J. CARPENTER, M.D., Professor of Medicine, Brown University, and The Miriam Hospital, Providence, Rhode Island
CIRO A. de QUADROS, M.D., M.P.H., Director, Division of Vaccines and Immunizations, Pan American Health Organization, Washington, D.C.
R. GORDON DOUGLAS, Jr., M.D., Princeton, New Jersey
LAWRENCE O. GOSTIN, J.D., LL.D. (Hon.), Codirector, Georgetown/Johns Hopkins Joint Program in Public Health and Law, and Professor of Law, Georgetown University, Washington, D.C.
M. CAROLYN HARDEGREE, M.D., Potomac, Maryland
SAMUEL L. KATZ, M.D., Wilburt C. Davison Professor and Chairman Emeritus, Duke University Medical Center, Durham, North Carolina
F. MARC LaFORCE, M.D., Director, Meningitis Vaccine Project, Program for Appropriate Technology in Health, Ferney-Voltaire, France
STANLEY A. PLOTKIN, M.D., Doylestown, Pennsylvania
GREGORY A. POLAND, M.D., Chief, Mayo Vaccine Research Group, Mayo Clinic and Foundation, Rochester, Minnesota
N. REGINA RABINOVICH, M.D., M.P.H., Director, Malaria Vaccine Initiative, Program for Appropriate Technology in Health, Rockville, Maryland
PHILIP K. RUSSELL, M.D., Special Advisor on Vaccine Development and Production, Office of Public Health Preparedness, Department of Health and Human Services, Washington, D.C.
RONALD J. SALDARINI, Ph.D., Mahwah, New Jersey
MARY E. WILSON, M.D., Chief of Infectious Diseases, Mount Auburn Hospital, and Associate Professor of Medicine, Harvard Medical School, Cambridge, Massachusetts

Staff

SUSAN THAUL, Ph.D., Study Director
SALEM FISSEHA, Research Assistant
RICHARD N. MILLER, M.D., M.P.H., Director, Medical Follow-up Agency
HEATHER O'MAONAIGH, M.A., Program Officer
PAMELA RAMEY-McCRAY, Administrative Assistant

Preface

In April 2000, the Institute of Medicine (IOM) of the National Academies convened an expert committee to advise the U.S. Army Medical Research and Materiel Command on the management of its vaccine research programs for the protection of U.S. military personnel against naturally occurring infectious disease threats. The charge to the committee focused on the army's Military Infectious Diseases Research Program and how it goes about its task of making available to the military new vaccines for the protection of warfighters against these constantly changing and emerging disease threats. That charge required the committee to examine broadly the process that the Department of Defense (DoD) uses to acquire and maintain the availability of vaccines. Doing so, the committee recognized that this process is too fragmented, too diffused, and too lacking in consolidation of its authority within a single responsible locus in DoD to operate efficiently and to be effective in meeting its critical mission. This report, the final product of the IOM Committee on a Strategy for Minimizing the Impact of Naturally Occurring Infectious Diseases of Military Importance: Vaccine Issues in the U.S. Military, details those findings as well as the information that was provided to the committee and that led it to reach these conclusions.

At the time that this report is being prepared for publication, the world is very different from the way it was 2 years earlier when the committee first convened. The terrorist attacks of September 11, 2001, and the subsequent mailing of lethally weaponized anthrax spores to members of the media and the U.S. Congress in the weeks that followed have forever altered the nation's sense of its vulnerability to terrorism in general and to the possibility of the intentional dissemination of potentially fatal infectious diseases in particular. These events have led to the proposal of enormous increases in the funding for infectious disease research, focused on biodefense, but certain to have significant spillover into the area of naturally transmitted infections. These new funds may answer, in whole or in part, one of the recommendations of this committee: that DoD substantially increase its budgetary support for infectious disease research and vaccine acquisition if it is to provide the protections required for the nation's warfighters in an increasingly complex and dangerous world.

However, DoD's interest in solving the problems with vaccine acquisition predated the events of September 11. Two important factors led to this growing concern over the functioning of vaccine acquisition efforts within DoD: (1) the awareness that the approach mandated by Congress for the development of countermeasures for biological warfare, the Joint Vaccine Acquisition Program, was failing to produce the vaccine products required and (2) the sudden loss from DoD's armamentarium of the very successful vaccine that DoD had previously developed for the prevention of adenovirus serotype 4 and 7 disease in military recruits. These events led the Deputy Secretary for Defense to commission a separate study and report shortly after the creation of this IOM committee. That committee, chaired by Franklin Top, Jr., addressed many issues that overlapped the issues that this committee was charged to address.

Although its contents were unknown to this committee for many months, the *Report on Biological Warfare Defense Vaccine Research and Development Programs*, through which DoD released the Top Report[1] to the public, ultimately presented conclusions very similar to those arrived at by this committee.

As explained in the pages that follow, this committee strongly believes that a full-fledged reorganization of DoD's priority-setting and vaccine acquisition processes will be required if the department is to fulfill its pledge to protect U.S. warfighters against vaccine-preventable infectious diseases. It believes that this is an issue of national security, inasmuch as infectious diseases have well-proven abilities to significantly degrade and compromise the operations of military forces. The major limitations, it believes, in making available safe and efficacious vaccines for the protection of forces have not been scientific in nature but, rather, revolve around problems of organization, management, and budgetary support.

Where possible, the committee has cited substantive data and evidence in support of these conclusions. In many instances, however, such hard data have simply not been available and the committee has had to draw on the past experiences and perceptions of its members, individuals who have spent their careers at the highest points of leadership in military research and development programs,

[1]Vaccine Study Panel. Department of Defense Acquisition of Vaccines Program: A Report to the Deputy Secretary of Defense from the Independent Panel of Experts, December 2000). In DoD 2001d. *Report on Biological Warfare Defense Vaccine Research and Development Programs*. Washington, DC: Department of Defense. [Online]. Available: http://www.defenselink.mil/pubs/ReportonBiologicalWarfareDefenseVaccineRDPrgras-July2001.pdf [accessed September 7, 2001].

the commercial vaccine industry, regulatory agencies, and academic infectious disease-related research and development communities.

The committee perceives with particular concern that the technology base and basic research activities of DoD are much narrower and limited in scope than they were in past decades, reflecting reductions in the numbers of military professional personnel, reductions in underlying budget support, and changes in program priorities. Although these trends are very difficult to document across the tens of years and the different military organizational structures that have evolved over time, none of the evidence that the committee reviewed refutes this belief. The committee believes that the technology base resides at the core of DoD's capacity to meet its mission in protecting U.S. warfighters against infectious disease threats. Its erosion should be a matter of national concern, and one that must be reversed through a sustained commitment of budget and personnel as the nation enters the twenty-first century.

To accomplish the task for which it convened this committee, IOM recognized that committee membership must include individuals with considerable expertise and experience in pharmaceutical research, development, and manufacturing. IOM found it impossible to recruit individuals with such backgrounds who do not also hold significant amounts of equity in the industry. IOM chose retired industry experts to minimize the potential conflict of interest. Committee members R. Gordon Douglas, Jr., Stanley A. Plotkin, and Ronald J. Saldarini each own significant stock and stock option holdings in pharmaceutical companies that are involved in vaccine development and manufacture. Their biographical summaries (included in Appendix C) illustrate the invaluable experience that they brought to this committee's work. At the first committee meeting, the Deputy Executive Officer of IOM conducted the required bias and conflict-of-interest discussion. All committee members were apprised of the points-of-view, experiences, and current activities of these committee members, as of all committee members, and were alerted to potential conflicts of interests. The vaccine manufacture section of Chapter 4 boldly presents a pharmaceutical industry view of the issues and labels it as such. The whole committee—aware of the source of advice—uniformly agreed with the analysis. It is my firm opinion that this judicious use of committee members whose potential conflicts of interest would ordinarily preclude their serving on IOM committees has been outstandingly successful and has served this committee and its sponsor well. The committee gained substantively from the experiences of those who have been close to commercial vaccine manufacture in the past, while it maintained its integrity by placing known biases and conflicts of interest on the table during discussions and also drawing heavily on the past experiences of other committee members in the regulation of vaccines and in both public and private vaccine development efforts.

Stanley M. Lemon, M.D.
Committee Chair

Acknowledgments

This project had a scope that included laboratory procedures and personnel; protection of human subjects in research; federal regulation; organizational design and management; financing; history; military operational readiness; political, military, and public health intelligence; vaccinology; and the study, prevention, and treatment of infectious diseases worldwide. Individual committee members are recognized experts in many of these fields, but all of them—and the study staff—needed education to introduce, review, or update areas in which they were less involved. For this education, we turned to people in DoD, FDA, CDC, NIH, and the vaccine industry, along with other colleagues. Appendix B contains the agenda listings from committee meeting open sessions; the invited presenters listed there shared a lot of information and perspective with the committee and staff. We thank them. Some information required staff pursuit by telephone, e-mail, and fax. Thanks are due to Dr. Kathryn Zoon and her colleagues Bette Goldman, Dr. Karen Midthun, and Loni Warren at FDA; Drs. Ellen Boudreau, Mark Kortepeter, and Phillip Pittman at USAMRIID; COL John Frazier Glenn and William Howell at USAMRMC; Dr. John Brundage, WRAIR; Dr. Francis E. Cole, Jr., JVAP; and Michael A. Paysan, Jr., Requirements and Acquisition Division, Joint Staff, Pentagon.

The recipient of the bulk of our requests for information was our sponsor representative COL Charles H. Hoke, Jr., director of the Military Infectious Diseases Research Program at USAMRMC through the core of the IOM project. He and his colleagues Drs. Lawrence Lightner and Rodney Michael fielded our questions through hundreds of e-mails, telephone calls and voice-mail messages, and perhaps a dozen in-person meetings. COL Hoke's task was large and his efforts to convey the scope of his concern for the direction of DoD in infectious diseases research, especially vaccine-related work, earned our respect. We greatly appreciate his efforts and those of his MIDRP colleagues. Thanks also to Peggy Nathan, MIDRP secretary-extraordinaire, whose resourcefulness we at times call upon for questions unrelated to this project.

Behind many great committee members are highly focused personal, administrative, or secretarial assistants. Over the last two years, we have relied on many and want to especially thank Deborah James and Denise Burrell for their work keeping us and our mail in touch with our committee chair, Dr. Stanley Lemon; three staffers at Mayo Clinic who relayed messages to and from Dr. Gregory Poland across the globe; Brenda Cole who did the same for Dr. Samuel Katz; and Grace Fries, who helped sort through Dr. Stanley Plotkin's numerous commitments to IOM activities.

We did not take all of the changes that our contract copyeditor Michael Hayes suggested. But just knowing that he would be editing the draft report made us write better. We thank him for his detailed and very thoughtful work.

The report was made possible by many staff members within the National Academies. Our thanks go to all of you, especially financial associate Andrea Cohen; Clyde Behney, Jennifer Bitticks, Carlos Orr, Jennifer Otten, and Bronwyn Schrecker in ORAC; Linda Kilroy in the Office of Contracts and Grants; Janice Mehler for the Report Review Committee; and Estelle Miller and Sally Stanfield at the National Academy Press. You each stepped up to move this project and report through to completion. Salem Fisseha, Richard Miller, Heather O'Maonaigh, Pamela Ramey-McCray, and I get our names on the final report. Others within the Medical Follow-up Agency helped us and the committee, whether by re-reading a paragraph to assure us that it said what we meant, offering (or withholding) candy or caffeine, managing guest support at committee meetings, or lending a hand when they saw we could use one. Thank you to Phillip Bailey, Harriet Crawford, Jihad Daghmash, Jane Durch, Rick Erdtmann, Reine Homawoo, Lois Joellenbeck, Karen Kazmerzak (who helped officially and well with this committee's interim letter report), William Page, Noreen Stevenson, and newcomer Laura Sivitz.

Finally, we acknowledge MG Lester Martinez-Lopez, USAMRMC commanding general, and COL David Vaughn, RAD1 director. They have stepped into their positions in time to receive this report; we thank them in advance for the time we anticipate they will give to the issues the IOM committee raises in this report.

Susan Thaul, Ph.D.
Study Director

Reviewers

This report has been reviewed in draft form by individuals chosen for their diverse perspectives and technical expertise, in accordance with procedures approved by the National Research Council's Report Review Committee. The purpose of this independent review is to provide candid and critical comments that will assist the institution in making its published report as sound as possible and to ensure that the report meets institutional standards for objectivity, evidence, and responsiveness to the study charge. The review comments and draft manuscript remain confidential to protect the integrity of the deliberative process. We wish to thank the following individuals for their review of this report:

DONALD S. BURKE, M.D., The Johns Hopkins University, Baltimore, Maryland
HENRY GRABOWSKI, Ph.D., Duke University, Durham, North Carolina
WILLIAM H. HABIG, Ph.D., Centocor, Inc., Malvern, Pennsylvania
BRUCE INNIS, M.D., GlaxoSmithKline Biologicals, Collegeville, Pennsylvania
CRAIG LLEWELLYN, M.D., M.P.H., MC USA COL (Ret.), Uniformed Services University of Health Sciences, Bethesda, Maryland
JACK MELLING, Ph.D., The Karl Landsteiner Institute, Vienna, Austria
FRANKLIN H. TOP, Jr., M.D., MedImmune, Inc., Gaithersburg, Maryland
MILTON C. WEINSTEIN, Ph.D., Harvard School of Public Health, Boston, Massachusetts

Although the reviewers listed above have provided many constructive comments and suggestions, they were not asked to endorse the conclusions or recommendations nor did they see the final draft of the report before its release. The review of this report was overseen by **Robert M. Chanock, M.D.,** National Institute of Allergy and Infectious Diseases, National Institutes of Health, and **Enriqueta C. Bond, Ph.D.,** Burroughs Wellcome Fund. Appointed by the Institute of Medicine and the National Research Council, they were responsible for making certain that an independent examination of this report was carried out in accordance with institutional procedures and that all review comments were carefully considered. Responsibility for the final content of this report rests entirely with the authoring committee and the institution.

Contents

Boxes, Figures, and Tables

BOXES

FIGURES

TABLES

Abbreviations and Acronyms

ACAT	acquisition category
AFEB	Armed Forces Epidemiological Board
AMEDD	Army Medical Department
ASA(ALT)	Assistant Secretary of the Army for Acquisition, Logistics, and Technology
ASBREM	Armed Services Biomedical Research, Evaluation and Management (Committee)
ASD(HA)	Assistant Secretary of Defense for Health Affairs
BSL	Biological Safety Level
CDC	Centers for Disease Control and Prevention
CRADA	Cooperative Research and Development Agreement
DHHS	Department of Health and Human Services
DoD	Department of Defense
DNA	deoxyribonucleic acid
DSCP	Defense Supply Center, Philadelphia
DTO	Defense Technology Objective
DUST	Dual-Use Science and Technology
ETEC	enterotoxigenic *Escherichia coli*
FDA	Food and Drug Administration
FHP	Force Health Protection

FOC	Future Operational Capability
FY	fiscal year
GAO	General Accounting Office
GOCO	government-owned, contractor-operated (manufacturing facility)
GSK	GlaxoSmithKline
HEV	hepatitis E virus
HIV	human immunodeficiency virus
IND	investigational new drug
IOM	Institute of Medicine
JTCG-2	Joint Technology Coordinating Group-2
JVAP	Joint Vaccine Acquisition Program
JWG	Joint Working Group
MEDCOM	U.S. Army Medical Command
MIDRP	Military Infectious Diseases Research Program
NAMRU-2	Navy Medical Research Unit 2
NIC	National Intelligence Council
NIH	National Institutes of Health
ORD	Operational Requirements Document
OSD	Office of the Secretary of Defense
RAD	Research Area Directorate
RDA	research, development, and acquisition
SIP	Special Immunizations Program
STEP	Science and Technology Evaluation Program
STO	Science and Technology Objective
TBE	tick-borne encephalitis
TRADOC	U.S. Army Training and Doctrine Command
TSI-GSD	The Salk Institute, Government Services Division
USAMMA	U.S. Army Medical Materiel Agency
USAMMDA	U.S. Army Medical Materiel Development Activity
USAMRAA	U.S. Army Medical Research Acquisition Activity
USAMRIID	U.S. Army Medical Research Institute of Infectious Diseases
USAMRMC	U.S. Army Medical Research and Materiel Command

USD(AT&L) Under Secretary of Defense for Acquisition, Technology, and Logistics

WRAIR Walter Reed Army Institute of Research

PROTECTING OUR FORCES

Executive Summary

PROJECT RATIONALE AND ORGANIZATION

Tremendous strides have been made in public health, the control of infectious diseases, and preventive medicine during the past century. Nevertheless, infectious agents remain a substantial threat to the operational capacity of U.S. military forces for three distinct reasons: (1) recruits continue to train in groups under crowded conditions, increasing the risk of spread of infectious agents; (2) deployed warfighters, whether on combat or peacekeeping missions, continue to come into contact with pathogens with which they have no prior experience and, therefore, against which they have no immunity; and (3) warfighters, along with others, face an increasing risk of the intentional use of weaponized infectious agents.

To review the process by which the U.S. military acquires vaccines to protect its warfighters against natural infectious disease threats, the Institute of Medicine (IOM) of the National Academies convened an expert committee, the Committee on a Strategy for Minimizing the Impact of Naturally Occurring Infectious Diseases of Military Importance: Vaccine Issues in the U.S. Military, in April 2000 to advise the U.S. Army Medical Research and Materiel Command (USAMRMC). This report is the final product of that IOM committee.

The charge to the committee was as follows:

> The committee will analyze available information, hold workshops and make specific recommendations on both technical and policy aspects regarding the Department of Defense vaccine strategy to combat infectious diseases. The issues include: (1) reviewing the problem of the naturally occurring infectious diseases threat to military operations; (2) defining and prioritizing the diseases of relevance to the U.S. military; (3) determining the status of vaccines available to protect military personnel; (4) examining the Military

> Infectious Diseases Research Program (MIDRP), with particular emphasis on current disease priorities, vaccine product development, and the role of the MIDRP not only within the framework of the overall Military Acquisition model, but also among other Federal government infectious disease programs; (5) reviewing the roles, if any, that the MIDRP should play in the licensure, manufacture, and distribution of vaccines against diseases of military importance, in the context of current interrelationships within DoD and among other federal agencies, industry, and university research activities; and (6) developing recommendations for a comprehensive strategy and doctrine that MIDRP and DoD could adopt to best use their resources to contribute toward the goal of effective development, licensure, production, stockpiling, distribution, and use of vaccines against naturally occurring diseases of military importance. Other issues regarding vaccine strategies against infectious diseases are likely to be brought to the attention of the committee by the DoD.

Based on their pre-committee experience, committee members believed that DoD's current administrative separation of acquisition processes for vaccines intended to protect against naturally occurring infectious diseases and acquisition of vaccines for defense against biological warfare is scientifically—and likely organizationally—unsound. The challenges of vaccine research and development are similar for both natural and weaponized sources of infectious agents. Moreover, some of the agents are the same and vaccines remain a preferred defense for both. Thus, although this report initially was intended to address only naturally occurring infectious disease threats, because vaccine policy concerns related to biodefense are inseparable from those dealing with naturally occurring disease threats, the committee has touched on issues pertaining to the acquisition of biodefense vaccines in this report when pertinent.

In addition, the committee has interpreted the charge's reference to "defining and prioritizing the diseases of relevance to the U.S. military" as a request to address how DoD should approach the issue of prioritization, rather than a request for the committee to offer a list of specific threats, diseases, or needed vaccine products.

The IOM committee met six times. It held open sessions at its first five meetings, hearing presentations from military personnel, those familiar with the vaccine industry, and infectious disease and vaccine experts. The committee used those briefings, its review of background material, and its members' past experiences and expertise in its deliberations.

The committee notes that various documents and individuals within government—including the Department of Defense (DoD)—and elsewhere use the term *acquisition* variably. For the purposes of its discussions, the committee defined *acquisition* as the process by which DoD ensures that appropriate vaccines are available for the protection of its forces. This process represents a continuum extending from the first recognition of need for a vaccine, through the setting of priorities, to the maintenance of a technology base. It includes internally conducted or externally contracted product-oriented research, advanced product development, and clinical studies leading to licensure. It also involves the establishment and maintenance of effective manufacturing facilities and, ultimately, the procurement (purchase) and stockpiling of vaccines for use by DoD for force protection.

This report contains four chapters. It begins with an historical overview of the influence of naturally occurring infectious diseases on U.S. military operations and the research that has been conducted in response to the threats posed by naturally occurring infectious diseases. Chapter 2 describes the role of USAMRMC in DoD—in particular its Research Area Directorate for Infectious Diseases that manages the Military Infectious Diseases Research Program (MIDRP)—in the acquisition of vaccines against infectious diseases; the chapter includes the committee's understanding of how current priorities emerge and the organizational context within which MIDRP operates. Chapter 3 describes current naturally occurring infectious disease threats and available vaccine countermeasures. In Chapter 4, the committee presents its recommendations in the context of its view of the limitations imposed by the current structure within DoD for managing the acquisition of vaccines against infectious diseases.

HISTORICAL OVERVIEW

A large body of historical literature describes the importance of infectious diseases in deciding the results of military campaigns. Napoleon ceased his advance in the eastern Mediterranean when faced with a plague outbreak in Jaffa. Florence Nightingale achieved fame by addressing the fundamental hygiene problems that had caused the extraordinarily high rates of injury-related gas gangrene during the Crimean War.

Up until World War II, deaths due to infectious diseases outnumbered those due to direct combat injuries (Gordon, 1958), and the potential remains for naturally occurring or intentionally disseminated infectious diseases to play a pivotal role in determining the outcomes of future conflicts. In addition, in recent years U.S. troops have frequently been deployed to geographic regions where there exist endemic infectious agents against which the U.S. military does not have immediately available suitable, safe, and effective vaccines or appropriate chemoprophylactic agents.

Military strategists have recognized the threat to military operations from infectious diseases since the beginning of the science of microbiology. The study of epidemics in military populations and the research done by military epidemiologists and microbiologists have led to major advances in public health and a better understanding of many infectious disease agents and their mechanisms of transmission. Two examples are Sir Ronald Ross's studies on the role of the *Anopheles* mosquito in the transmission of malaria and Walter Reed's observations on the role of the *Aedes aegypti* mosquito as a vector for the spread of yellow fever.

Vaccines have served as a key mode of preventing infections among America's military forces since General George Washington ordered the systematic variolation of the Continental Army to protect the nascent nation's soldiers from smallpox.

VACCINE MISSION AND PROCEDURES OF USAMRMC

USAMRMC, a subordinate command of the U.S. Army Medical Command, is charged with solving medical problems and providing medical product solutions to the U.S. armed forces. Among these solutions are vaccines. USAMRMC's primary goal is to protect and sustain the health of the warfighter. Its website states that it is responsible for medical research, product development, technology assessment and rapid prototyping, medical logistics management, health facility planning, and medical information management and technology.

USAMRMC estimates its fiscal year 2002 infectious diseases research funding (both vaccine-related and other projects) at approximately $63 million, not including its congressionally mandated and separately funded HIV-related activities.[1] With activities throughout the United States and overseas, USAMRMC works from its headquarters, six research laboratory commands, and six administrative commands or directorates. The Army assigns approximately 4,600 military and civilian personnel to these units. As part of its medical research and development charge, USAMRMC manages research as well as product development related to, among other things, vaccines and therapeutic agents aimed at preventing and controlling naturally occurring infectious diseases that are perceived to threaten the operational effectiveness of the armed forces. However, USAMRMC does not manage the advanced development of vaccines against weaponized infectious agents; DoD assigns that mission to the Joint Vaccine Acquisition Program.

Despite its role in vaccine acquisition, USAMRMC is not formally involved in determining DoD policy for vaccine use. The Office of the Assistant Secretary of Defense for Health Affairs establishes and implements policies relating to the health care services to be offered to the members of the U.S. armed forces. The civilian expert members of the Armed Forces Epidemiological Board, a standing scientific advisory committee under the executive agency of the Army, serve as scientific advisers to DoD and address issues such as disease control, health maintenance, and disease prevention, including the use of vaccines.

It is noteworthy that USAMRMC is but one of many players in the current process in DoD by which the earliest recognition of a military medical problem leads to the development and acquisition of a licensed vaccine that is available for use by military personnel. Proposals for the acquisition of new vaccine

[1] Dollar estimates are shown in more detail in Table 2-1 of the full report.

products for use by military personnel must pass through a complex series of priority-setting and budgeting processes and through the hands of various USAMRMC managers, as well as numerous DoD stakeholders outside USAMRMC. Within USAMRMC, the Research Area Directorate for Infectious Diseases, through MIDRP, which involves all military services, coordinates the early stages of research and development; and the U.S. Army Medical Materiel Development Activity works on the advanced development of specific products. DoD's research efforts are facilitated by a number of cooperative agreements that are used to secure relationships with vaccine manufacturers, academic institutions, other governments, and U.S. government agencies other than DoD.

Within DoD, operations and maintenance funding for the purchase and maintenance of acquired medical products (including vaccines) is managed separately from the research and development funding for vaccine-related research and development. Vaccine products recommended for use for the protection of new recruits or for general use among all members of the armed services are procured with funds for medical care (Defense Health Care). The USAMRMC commanding general has no authority in this process. Some vaccines recommended for use in specific deployments do, however, fall within the nominal authority of the USAMRMC through the U.S. Army Medical Materiel Agency.

DoD administers 17 different vaccines for the prevention of infectious diseases among military personnel. The vaccines are administered to military personnel, where appropriate, on the basis of military occupation, the location of the deployment, and mission requirements.

DISCUSSION

Protecting the health of military personnel is essential to national security. Vaccines are often the most cost-effective way to protect individuals from infectious diseases, but their value is easily overlooked both within the civilian public health sector and within the military. The committee believes that DoD must assign a much higher priority to vaccine acquisition than it does now. In sifting through the evidence and hearing from a considerable number of those who are directly involved with vaccine acquisition, the committee came to realize that the current DoD vaccine acquisition process does not take sufficient account of the fact that vaccines are complex systems and not simply commodities that can be specified, procured, and placed on the shelf for future use.

Much care and forethought are required for the development and initial acquisition of vaccines. The need for attention does not end once vaccines are licensed and made available to the military. DoD must continuously monitor the status of licensed vaccines and needs to have the ability to modify vaccines, including manufacturing processes and the facilities in which vaccines are produced, as regulatory agencies seek changes in the light of new scientific knowledge or in an effort to ensure product safety. To do this efficiently, the committee concluded that a single authority needs to oversee both the advanced development and the procurement of vaccines, among other parts of the process, lest a licensed product be lost from the armamentarium because of an inability to support further refinement and development of the vaccine. An example of DoD's lack of attention to the systems aspects of a protective vaccine is the loss of the vaccines against adenovirus serotypes 4 and 7 and the increased rates of respiratory disease that occurred among basic trainees when the vaccines were no longer available. A consolidation of authority across the entire spectrum of vaccine acquisition activities would help to solve this problem, as laid out in the specific recommendations that follow. At the same time, the committee concluded that the current duplication of management structures—for acquisition of vaccines for protection against biological warfare and for those for protection from naturally occurring infectious diseases—makes little sense. This is because many pathogens that may be used for biological warfare also occur naturally, and because the scientific, technical, manufacturing, and stockpiling issues that both programs face are so very similar.

After reviewing the available evidence, the committee concluded that DoD's vaccine acquisition procedures, coupled with its complex annual budgeting process, significantly hamper its vaccine acquisition activities and thwart effective coordination with the vaccine industry. These limitations prevent DoD from developing important vaccines. They also cause instability in essential vaccine-related research programs and result in an inability to have available for immediate use those vaccines that are critical for the protection of military personnel. Such an inefficient acquisition process puts military readiness at risk. Some militarily important vaccines are not available, in whole or in part, because of poorly aligned acquisition processes and an inadequate commitment of financial resources rather than uncleared scientific or technological hurdles.

DoD's approach to vaccines originates with the best intentions, involves skilled individuals, millions (but not sufficient millions) of dollars in funding, and intricate planning. Still, the committee believes that limitations in the acquisition process make the path from basic research to the procurement and use of vaccines both inefficient financially and cumbersome, resulting in occasional failure (as in the case of the adenovirus type 4 and 7 vaccines) and unacceptable delays (in the case of the anthrax vaccine) in vaccine acquisition. This approach risks the success of military operations and the health of personnel, and potentially places national security in jeopardy.

RECOMMENDATIONS

The committee's recommendations, presented in Box ES-1, cover four broad aspects of the acquisition process: organization, authority, and responsibility; program and budget; manufacturing; and regulatory status of special-use vaccines. Chapter 4 of the report discusses each recommendation and provides the avail-

BOX ES-1
Committee Recommendations

Organization, Authority, and Responsibility

The committee recommends that the Department of Defense:

1. Combine all DoD vaccine acquisition responsibilities under a single DoD authority that includes the entire spectrum of responsibility—from potential threat definition through research and development, advanced product development, clinical trials, licensure, manufacture, procurement, and continued maintenance of manufacturing practice standards and regulatory compliance.

2. Consolidate infrastructure, funding, and personnel for DoD acquisition programs for biodefense and naturally occurring infectious disease vaccines.

3. Ensure that there is an effective, ongoing senior advisory group—one providing perspectives from both within and outside of DoD—to assess program priorities and accomplishments, to act as a proponent for vaccines and other infectious disease countermeasures, and to maintain active relationships with current science and technology leaders in academic, government, and corporate sectors.

Program and Budget

The committee recommends that the Department of Defense:

4. Provide budget resources commensurate with the task.

5. Actively encourage the development, distribution, and use of a well-defined and validated research priority-setting mechanism, which could involve prioritized, weighted lists of infectious disease threats and formal scenario-planning exercises. To do so requires infectious diseases surveillance and the collection and synthesis of epidemiologic information.

6. Include programming goals that ensure greater strength and continuity in the science and technology base across the full spectrum of infectious disease threats, including research related to the epidemiology of infectious diseases, the nature of protective immunity, and both early and advanced vaccine product development.

7. Leverage DoD research efforts by building greater interactions and an effective formalized coordinating structure that links DoD research to vaccine development activities carried out by the Department of Health and Human Services and other public and private groups.

Manufacturing

The committee recommends that the Department of Defense:

8. Work toward manufacturing arrangements that ensure consistent vaccine availability by addressing long-term commitment, predictable volumes and prices, indemnification, and intellectual property issues. These arrangements should include consideration of vaccine-specific, government partnerships with individual private manufacturers, a private manufacturer consortium, and government-owned, contractor-operated vaccine-production facilities.

Regulatory Status of Special-Use Vaccines

The committee recommends that the Department of Defense:

9. Vigorously seek a new paradigm for the regulation of special-use vaccines that remain in Investigational New Drug status with the Food and Drug Administration without reasonable prospects of licensure under current rules, ensuring demonstration of the safety and efficacy of these products commensurate with their anticipated use.

able supporting evidence and a description of the committee's reasoning that led to each recommendation.

CONCLUSION

Partly because of the past success of DoD research programs, the public and even DoD personnel outside of the medical sphere know little about the contributions of the military's infectious disease programs or the threats that its products have ameliorated. By creating a single vaccine authority with a credible advisory board and with budgetary authority and responsibility extending across the broad continuum of the vaccine acquisition cycle, from setting priorities to stockpiling of licensed products, DoD would enhance not only the effectiveness but also the visibility of its vaccine program. The creation of such an authority would also improve the likelihood that the vaccine acquisition process would be provided with a budget that is sufficient to accomplish its mission. It is a mission of enormous importance. Immunization is often the most effective means of preventing infectious diseases, in either civilian or military populations, and whether caused by naturally encountered infectious agents or purposeful exposures related to bioterrorism or biological warfare.

In summary, DoD's vaccine acquisition program, despite its distinguished history, diffuses responsibility and is inadequately funded; therefore, it cannot produce the effort required to respond to a task that has been made more urgent by the continuing emergence of new natural infectious disease threats and growing recognition of the risks of bioterrorism and biological warfare.

The committee urges DoD to work more aggressively with decision makers in the U.S. Congress and in the executive branch to recognize that infectious disease agents—whether they occur naturally or are weaponized as agents of biological warfare or terror—threaten military operations and, therefore and implicitly, the welfare of the nation. Decision makers must recognize (1) the past, imminent, and possible future successes of vaccines in minimizing those threats; (2) the strong track records and reputations of military research programs in developing vaccines used by the U.S. military as well as in civilian settings; (3) the contributions that DoD's medical research efforts make to foreign policy and national security; (4) the threats to continued vaccine development and the ultimate availability of vaccines that are posed by organizational and fiscal limits; and, consequently, (5) the need for adequate, stable funding and strong management authority. Such changes would allow DoD to optimally advance and exploit the technology available for vaccine development, and to provide the best possible protection of the nation's armed forces against infectious diseases.

1

Introduction and History

NATURALLY OCCURRING INFECTIOUS DISEASES IN THE U.S. MILITARY

Despite the tremendous strides that have been made in public health, the control of infectious diseases, and preventive medicine during the past century, infectious agents remain a substantial threat to the operational capacity of military forces at the onset of the new millennium for three distinct reasons: (1) new recruits are trained in groups under crowded conditions, increasing the risk of spread of infectious agents; (2) warfighters, as a result of deployments, may come into contact with pathogens with which they have no prior experience and, therefore, no immunity; and (3) warfighters, along with others, may face the intentional use of weaponized infectious agents.

Until World War II, deaths due to infectious diseases outnumbered those due to direct combat injuries (Gordon, 1958). A large body of historical literature exists describing the importance of infectious diseases in deciding the results of military campaigns. Napoleon ceased his advance in the eastern Mediterranean when faced with a plague outbreak in Jaffa. Florence Nightingale achieved fame by addressing the fundamental hygiene problems that had caused the extraordinarily high rates of injury-related gas gangrene during the Crimean War. She, along with William Farr, compared mortality data for soldiers against a civilian standard. Finding that men of military age in England and Wales had an annual mortality of 9.2/1,000 compared to one of 35.0/1,000 for servicemen, Farr and Nightingale showed that most of the excess mortality among members of the military was due to contagious diseases and crowding (Curtin, 1989). Modern conflicts have been no different, as evidenced by the experiences of the Axis forces with infectious hepatitis during the North African campaign and the wide variety of infectious diseases that affected American warfighters in Vietnam. Although the use of vaccines against plague and cholera significantly minimized the incidence of those diseases among U.S troops in Vietnam (Ellenbogen, 1982; Ognibene, 1987), diseases for which vaccines were not available—for example, leptospirosis, meliodosis, and shigellosis—were prevalent (Ognibene, 1987). Even in recent years, U.S. troops have been deployed to geographic regions where there exist endemic infectious disease agents against which the U.S. military does not have immediately available either suitable, safe, and effective vaccines or appropriate chemoprophylactic agents. Infectious diseases continue to contribute substantially to morbidity during deployments, as shown in Figure 1-1.

The severity of the threat to military operations from infectious diseases has been recognized since the beginning of the science of microbiology and has prompted a substantial body of military research on the subject and many advances in public health. A better understanding of many infectious agents and their mechanisms of transmission have come from careful studies of epidemics in military populations and from research done by military epidemiologists and microbiologists. Two examples are Sir Ronald Ross's studies on the role of the

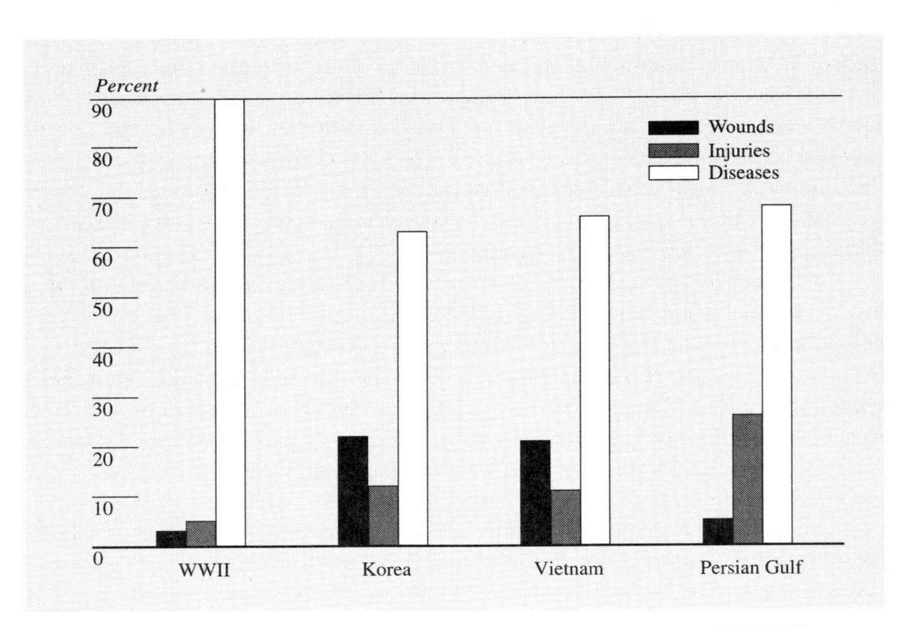

FIGURE 1-1 U.S. Army hospital admissions during war. SOURCE: NIC (2000).

Anopheles mosquito in the transmission of malaria and Walter Reed's observations on the role of the *Aedes aegypti* mosquito as a vector for the spread of yellow fever. Another example is offered by the classic studies of infectious and serum hepatitis (due to hepatitis A and hepatitis B viruses, respectively) that were carried out by the U.S. Army during World War II and that clearly delineated the separate and unrelated nature of these infectious agents and the diseases that they caused (Paul and Gardner, 1960).

Immunization has long served as a key mode of prevention of infections in military populations. General George Washington ordered the first systematic immunization effort among American forces when he directed the variolation of Revolutionary War soldiers serving in the Continental Army to protect them from smallpox (Bayne-Jones, 1968). Table 1-1 summarizes important advances in the control of militarily important infectious diseases that have resulted in part or in whole from the activities of the Army Medical Department. The list is a veritable history of public health advances and testifies to the key role that military scientists and epidemiologists have played not only in keeping soldiers healthy but also in contributing to improvements in the general public health.

Infectious Disease Threats During Recent Deployments of U.S. Military Forces

U.S. troops must be prepared to be deployed anywhere in the world, often on very short notice, whether it is for actual combat, for a training exercise, or to serve as peacekeepers. Given the political instabilities in many parts of the world, U.S. warfighters must be ready to be deployed into environments where the risk of exposure to infectious diseases may be significant. Deployments occur in areas with widely different climates and very different ecological and demographic settings, including, within just the past 10 years, the Caribbean, the Middle East, South-Central Asia, and the Western Pacific. As this report is being drafted, U.S. warfighters are deployed in Afghanistan and are being sent in increasing numbers to the Philippines, neither of which would have readily been predicted as a location for deployment at the time that this study was commissioned. Predicting the nature and magnitude of infectious disease risks in advance of deployments may not always be possible, but maintaining a high degree of awareness is mandatory, given the lessons of history and the clear benefit-to-cost ratio. Table 1-2 summarizes the scope of infectious disease risks that U.S. troops have faced during deployments since 1900.

U.S. forces will face these risks, as well as new ones, as long as they are deployed into unfamiliar environments. Global military disease surveillance activities must continue to furnish information about these risks so that preventive strategies can be developed in the event of deployment (Ognibene, 1987).

TABLE 1-1 Historical Highlights in the Control of U.S. Military Infectious Diseases by Vaccines

Year	Event
1777	Members of Continental Army inoculated with the variola virus to prevent smallpox
1812	Cowpox immunization replaced variolation for prevention of smallpox in troops
1909	Typhoid vaccine developed
1927	Chloroform-treated single-dose rabies vaccine for dogs developed through work done in the Philippines
1940s	Dengue virus types 1 and 2 isolated; first experiments begun with dengue vaccine
1940s	Tetanus toxoid and diphtheria toxoid shown to be highly effective in preventing wound-induced tetanus and diphtheria infections
1941	Armed Forces Epidemiological Board established; commissions established to deal with influenza, hepatitis, encephalitis, and other diseases that threatened the war effort; vaccine-related activities included conducting research and providing immunization policy advice
1942	Influenza vaccine developed and used for mass immunization of military forces
1942	Yellow fever vaccine used in large numbers of military personnel; hepatitis B virus contamination of serum causes a large common-source outbreak of jaundice
1944	Smallpox vaccine licensed
1944	Troops stationed in Okinawa, Japan, immunized against Japanese encephalitis
1950s	Discovery that adenovirus types 3, 4, and 7 cause most cases of acute respiratory diseases in recruits; adenovirus vaccine research and development initiated
1950s	Anthrax vaccine developed
1960s	Outbreaks of meningococcal meningitis on military posts stimulated the study of meningococcal infection and the development of vaccines against meningococcal groups A, C, Y, and W-135
1960s	Plague vaccine proven effective in Vietnam
1960s	Malaria vaccine program initiated (protection from bite of radiated mosquitoes shown)

Year	Event
1965–1969	INDs* filed for vaccines against Venezuelan equine encephalitis, tularemia, eastern equine encephalitis, and Rift Valley fever
1970s	Development and testing of an oral typhoid vaccine
1970s	Prototype vaccines against Russian spring-summer encephalitis and tick-borne encephalitis made at Walter Reed Army Institute of Research (WRAIR)
1970s	Live attenuated dengue virus vaccine strains developed; INDs filed
1970	Anthrax vaccine licensed
1972–1975	INDs filed for Q fever vaccine and live attenuated Venezuelan equine encephalitis virus vaccine
1980	Adenovirus vaccines licensed for use in military populations, leading to nearly complete control of epidemic respiratory diseases in recruits
1984–1986	INDs filed for vaccines against western equine encephalitis, Argentine hemorrhagic fever, Venezuelan equine encephalitis, and chikungunya virus
1985	Efficacy of Japanese encephalitis vaccine demonstrated in Thailand; licensure application coordinated by U.S. Army Medical Materiel Development Activity; license granted by Food and Drug Administration
1985–1986	Hepatitis A vaccine developed and tested by WRAIR
1986	WRAIR classification of human immunodeficiency virus infections published
1987	Manufacturing technology for hepatitis A vaccine transferred from WRAIR to a commercial manufacturer; vaccine licensed in 1995
1991	IND filed for Rift Valley fever vaccine
1996	Recombinant circumsporozoite malaria vaccine developed by the U.S. Army and an industrial partner shown to be protective in human volunteers
1997	First successful vaccine against Shigella developed, produced, and tested
1998	First DNA vaccine against malaria administered to humans

* An investigational new drug (IND) application is filed when a product is ready for human testing. Specific regulations govern the use of IND products (Investigational new drug application [IND]. 21 CFR § 312.20–312.21, subpart B [2001]; also see discussion in Chapter 3).

SOURCE: Modified from Hoke (2000a).

TABLE 1-2 Major Infectious Disease Threats for Which There Were No Licensed Vaccines at the Time of Deployments and Overseas Exercises

Place	Year	Infectious Disease Threat
Bosnia	1996	Diarrhea, hemorrhagic fever renal syndrome, mycoplasma infection, tick-borne encephalitis
Haiti	1994	Dengue, malaria
Somalia	1993	Dengue, diarrhea, malaria
Botswana	1992	African tick typhus, malaria
Saudi Arabia, Kuwait, and Iraq	1990–1991	Botulism,* diarrhea, enterotoxigenic *Escherichia coli* infection, leishmaniasis, sandfly fever
Egypt	1983	Diarrhea
Lebanon	1982	Diarrhea
Vietnam	1959–1975	Dengue, diarrhea, hepatitis, Japanese encephalitis, leptospirosis, malaria, melioidosis, murine typhus, scrub typhus, sexually transmitted diseases (STDs; especially gonorrhea)
Lebanon	1958	Diarrhea
Korea	1950–1953	Hepatitis, Japanese encephalitis, Korean hemorrhagic fever, malaria, STDs (especially gonorrhea)
World War II, Pacific	1941–1946	Dengue, diarrhea, filariasis, Japanese encephalitis, malaria, meningitis, schistosomiasis, scrub typhus, STDs
World War II, North Africa	1940–1941	Diarrhea, hepatitis, malaria, meningitis, sandfly fever
World War I	1917–1918	Diarrhea, influenza, meningitis, pneumonia, tetanus, typhus, wound infections
Cuba	1900	Malaria, typhoid, yellow fever

*The available product was not licensed and was administered as an investigational new drug.

SOURCE: Modified from Hoke (2000a).

SETTING PRIORITIES FOR MILITARY MEDICAL RESEARCH THROUGH THE TWENTIETH CENTURY

Since the end of the Cold War, the nature of U.S. military operations has changed. The troop deployments of today are smaller, faster, more diverse, and more diffuse, and they entail more frequent endeavors than military engagements of yore. This shift in activity has been accompanied by a change in operating strategy, including adoption by DoD of a fundamental Force Health Protection (FHP) tenet. Central to FHP is the concept that "the most valuable, most complex weapons system the U.S. military will ever field are its soldiers, sailors, airmen, and marines. These human weapon systems require lifecycle support and maintenance. . ." (JSLD, 1999, p. 2). Preventive medicine is a key component of FHP. Vaccination is, in turn, a key component of infectious disease prevention.

DoD interest in infectious disease prevention has been reinforced by Presidential Decision Directive NSTC (National Science and Technology Council)-7, which calls for DoD involvement in stepped-up U.S. efforts to address emerging infectious diseases (NSTC, 1996) and by National Intelligence Council (NIC) recognition that infectious diseases pose a threat to national security. "New and reemerging infectious diseases will pose a rising global health threat and will complicate U.S. and global security over the next 20 years," NIC concludes in its January 2000 National Intelligence Estimate. "These diseases will endanger U.S. citizens at home and abroad, threaten U.S. armed forces deployed overseas, and exacerbate social and political instability in key countries and regions in which the United States has significant interests" (NIC, 2000, p. 5). Similar sentiments are echoed by many (IOM, 1992; Kassalow, 2001; Kelley, 1999). DoD's responsibility for the protection of military and civilian populations alike compels its interest in infectious disease prevention and, by extension, vaccines.

History

Although many things have changed during the more than century-long history of the Army Medical Department's research and development efforts, the Army Medical Department's goal has stayed remarkably constant: highly focused research and product development efforts designed to mitigate the impacts of infectious diseases on military operations. In 1893, Army Surgeon General George M. Sternberg established the Army Medical School, now the Walter Reed Army Institute of Research, which has since served as a center for the Army's medical research efforts (Engelman and Joy, 1975). At the end of the nineteenth and early in the twentieth century, for example, the department addressed the infectious disease threats that caused the greatest numbers of casualties during the Civil and Spanish–American Wars. It was not difficult for Sternberg, Reed, and colleagues to know which diseases they should focus on: the well-recorded burden of typhoid fever, yellow fever, malaria, dengue, and diarrhea on military operations and medical care systems had made the priorities obvious.

As late as the Vietnam War, the surgeons general of the armed services used similar data—material that emerged from the military health care system and the records of the influence of infectious diseases on the effectiveness of military units—in setting priorities. In coming to their decisions, the surgeons general regularly relied on advice from the Armed Forces Epidemiological Board, a group of civilian experts who, for decades, considerably influenced both disease prevention policies and military medical research priorities.

Not surprisingly, research needs have differed from war to war. World War II generated intense research and development efforts on a wide range of infectious diseases. In contrast, the Korean War generated an upsurge in more focused research on malaria, arboviruses, and hemorrhagic fevers. The Vietnam War experience resulted in focused attention on malaria, viral hepatitis, dengue, scrub typhus, murine typhus, leptospirosis, bacterial diarrheas, and plague.

How Current Priorities Emerge

Ironically, the considerable success of these efforts has complicated the management of military medical research and development efforts to control infectious diseases. For example, many infectious disease threats of the past are no longer as dangerous as they once were. In the most recent deployments, military preventive medicine measures such as the provision of safe water and food and the use of vaccines, chemoprophylaxis, and vector control measures—along with favorable combat conditions—have kept the numbers of casualties from infectious diseases low. Therefore, decision makers often must rely on estimates of the potential of newly emerging infectious diseases, the extent of emerging microbial resistance to chemoprophylatic agents, and the regionally important illnesses for which epidemiologic information may be incomplete and for which proven vaccines or medical countermeasures do not exist.

At the same time, funding decisions and the administrative processes by which priorities are set must wend their way through increasingly complex layers of bureaucracy. This process is described in detail in Chapter 2.

Despite historic successes, in recent years DoD vaccine acquisition efforts have at times been troubled. This is best exemplified by the loss of the availability of adenovirus, plague, and anthrax vaccines. Although the circumstances contributing to the loss of the availability of each vaccine differ, each case illustrates the vulnerabilities inherent in the vaccine acquisition system.

In the 1960s and 1970s widespread adenovirus infections, especially those due to serotypes 4 and 7, plagued the armed forces basic training facilities throughout each winter-spring respiratory virus season, resulting in major morbidity and some mortality, overtaxed and overcrowded hospital facilities, and the loss of significant amounts of time from basic training as a result of recurrent explosive outbreaks. As a result, military research efforts were directed toward the development of serotype-specific vaccines. These vaccines were shown to be highly effective in trials in the 1960s and early 1970s (Edmondson et al., 1966; Top et al., 1971) and became licensed in 1980. Administration of these oral, live encapsulated adenovirus type 4 and 7 vaccines to recruits on the first day of their arrival at a base rendered the outbreaks a thing of the past. After 25 years of successful use, discussions between DoD and the manufacturer failed to produce an agreement concerning improvements to the manufacturing facility that were required by the Food and Drug Administration (FDA). The sole manufacturer of the adenovirus vaccines stopped producing them in 1996, and the stock was totally depleted by mid-1999. Subsequently, adenovirus illness reemerged as a major cause of illness and hospitalization among new trainees (Gray et al., 1999; McNeill et al., 1999; Sanchez et al., 2001). Virus studies in 1999 and 2000 revealed that 82 percent of the infections were again due to types 4 and 7. Thousands of trainees have been affected, and as a result, many recruits must repeat their training because of time lost due to illness (Gray et al., 2000). Three basic training facilities found their infirmary and hospital facilities overwhelmed and were forced to seek other accommodations for trainees requiring inpatient care. The deaths of at least two previously healthy recruits have been attributed to vaccine-preventable adenovirus infections (CDC, 2001). This committee issued a letter report to the Commanding General of the U.S. Army Medical Research and Materiel Command on November 6, 2000, to urge action to restore the availability and production of adenovirus vaccines (IOM, 2000a). The letter report is reprinted as Appendix A to this report.

The availability of the plague vaccine has also been interrupted. Plague vaccine, first manufactured in the United States by Miles Inc. in 1942 (IOM, 1993), has mostly military but some commercial applications. In 1990, Greer Laboratories took over production of the vaccine (AFEB, 1999). In a September 22, 1997 warning letter to Greer Laboratories, FDA outlined several significant deviations from FDA production guidelines in the manufacture of the company's plague vaccine (FDA, 1997c). Greer Laboratories discontinued the vaccine in 1998 because "FDA requirements for further testing and validation of the product could not be financially justified, and DoD was not able to fund further studies" (Greer Laboratories, 2001). Currently, plague vaccine is not available to protect U.S. forces.

The anthrax vaccine, adsorbed, also was available in only limited supply to the U.S. military due to regulatory compliance issues. The license to manufacture the vaccine was granted to one manufacturer, the Michigan Department of Public Health, in 1970. Ownership of the facility was transferred to Michigan Biologics Products Institute (MBPI) in 1995 and in 1998 the facility was sold to BioPort. Bioport retains the sole license to manufacture the anthrax vaccine. In March 1997, FDA issued MBPI a Notice of Intent to Revoke after routine inspection of the manufacturing facility by FDA in November 1996 revealed "significant deviations from the Food, Drug, and Cosmetic Act, FDA's regulations and the standards of MBPI's license" for the manufacture of blood-derived products and bacterial vaccines (FDA, 1997a; Zoon, 2000, p. 12). Although production of the vaccine had resumed in 1999 (IOM, 2002), BioPort had not been able to release any new lots of the vaccine without further inspections and official FDA approval, significantly restricting the availability of the vaccine to the U.S. military. BioPort upgraded its facilities to comply with FDA standards and on December 27, 2001 and January 31, 2002, respectively, FDA approved a license supplement for the renovations to BioPort's facility and an additional supplement for the contractor-operated filling site (BioPort Corporation, 2002; IOM, 2002). The approval of the two license supplements has made the vaccine available—once again—to the U.S. military.

ABOUT THIS REPORT

In April 2000, the Institute of Medicine (IOM) of the National Academies convened an expert committee to advise the U.S. Army Medical Research and Materiel Command on the management of research and development efforts related to naturally occurring infectious disease threats to members of the U.S. military, in particular, the acquisition of vaccines to prevent these diseases. This report is the final product of that group, the Committee on a Strategy for Minimizing the Impact of Naturally Occurring Infectious Diseases of Military Importance: Vaccine Issues in the U.S. Military.

The charge to the committee was as follows:

> The committee will analyze available information, hold workshops and make specific recommendations on both technical and policy aspects regarding the Department of Defense vaccine strategy to combat infectious diseases. The issues include: (1) reviewing the problem of the naturally occurring infectious diseases threat to military operations; (2) defining and prioritizing the diseases of relevance to the U.S. military; (3) determining the status of vaccines available to protect military personnel; (4) examining the Military Infectious Diseases Research Program (MIDRP), with particular emphasis on current disease priorities, vaccine product development, and the role of the MIDRP not only within the framework of the overall Military Acquisition model, but also among other Federal government infectious disease programs; (5) reviewing the roles, if any, that the MIDRP should play in the licensure, manufacture, and distribution of vaccines against diseases of military importance, in the context of current interrelationships within DoD and among other federal agencies, industry, and university research activities; and (6) developing recommendations for a comprehensive strategy and doctrine that MIDRP and DoD could adopt to best use their resources to contribute toward the goal of effective development, licensure, production, stockpiling, distribution, and use of vaccines against naturally occurring diseases of military importance. Other issues regarding vaccine strategies against infectious diseases are likely to be brought to the attention of the committee by the DoD.

The IOM committee met six times, holding open sessions at its first five meetings and hearing presentations from military personnel, those familiar with the vaccine industry, and infectious disease and vaccine experts. The committee used those briefings, its review of background material, and its members' experiences and expertise in its deliberations. As the committee began its work, it made two interpretive decisions about the charge it had been given.

On the basis of their experiences before they became members of the committee, committee members believed that DoD's current administrative separation of research and development efforts related to vaccines against naturally occurring infectious diseases and vaccines against biological agents that may be weaponized was scientifically—and likely organizationally—unsound. The challenges of vaccine-related research and development are similar for vaccines against both natural and weaponized infectious agents. Moreover, many of the agents both occur naturally and can be used as biological weapons, and vaccination remains the preferred type of medical defense against both types of threats. Thus, although this report was initially intended to address only naturally occurring infectious disease threats, because vaccine policy concerns related to biodefense are inseparable from those dealing with naturally occurring infectious disease threats, in this report, when pertinent, the committee has touched on issues addressing the acquisition of vaccines against biological agents that may be weaponized.

In addition, the committee has interpreted the charge's reference to "defining and prioritizing the diseases of relevance to the U.S. military" as a request to address how DoD might approach the issue of prioritization rather than a request for the committee to offer a list of specific threats, diseases, or needed vaccine products.

Report Organization

This report, presented in four chapters, began with an historical overview of the influence of naturally occurring infectious diseases on U.S. military operations and the research that has been conducted in response to these threats. In Chapter 2, the committee describes the current role of the U.S. Army Medical Research and Materiel Command in infectious disease-related research and development and vaccine acquisition, including the committee's understanding of how current priorities emerge and the organizational context within which MIDRP operates within DoD. Chapter 3 describes current naturally occurring infectious disease threats and the available vaccine countermeasures. In Chapter 4, the committee presents it recommendations in the context of its view of the limitations imposed by the current structure for managing infectious disease-related research and development and vaccine acquisition within DoD.

2

Resources, Responsibilities, and Dynamics in the Military's Vaccine Mission

The process of acquiring and maintaining the availability of vaccines for use by the U.S. military is supported by an intricate, multitiered, and continually changing Department of Defense (DoD) organizational structure that encompasses military and civilian elements and that operates within the respective branches of the armed forces. The U.S. Congress has designated the U.S. Army as the lead agent for DoD infectious diseases research.[1] The steps leading to the availability of a vaccine that protects military personnel against an infectious disease include identification of a need, research, development, testing, production, evaluation, regulatory compliance, and procurement. In this chapter, the committee describes these steps and associated DoD organizational components to the extent that they are relevant to its charge.

Over the course of this study, this committee has come to appreciate, though not completely comprehend, the complex and convoluted nature of the system by which DoD acquires vaccines. The complexity of this system is, perhaps, best depicted in Figure 2-1.

A more detailed description of this process—as it is understood by the committee—follows.

VACCINE MISSION OF THE U.S. ARMY MEDICAL RESEARCH AND MATERIEL COMMAND

The U.S. Army Medical Research and Materiel Command (USAMRMC), a subordinate command of the U.S. Army Medical Command (MEDCOM)

[1]Department of Defense Appropriations Act, 1982, P.L. 97-114 (1981).

(Figure 2-2), is charged with solving medical problems and providing the armed forces with solutions to these problems in the form of medical products; among these solutions are vaccines. USAMRMC's primary goal is to protect and sustain the health of the warfighter (USAMRMC, 2001a). To accomplish this goal, USAMRMC is "responsible for medical research, product development, technology assessment and rapid prototyping, medical logistics management, health facility planning, and medical information management and technology" (USAMRMC, 2001a).

With activities throughout the United States and overseas, USAMRMC comprises its headquarters, six research laboratory commands, and six[2] administrative commands or directorates. These laboratory and administrative commands are named as USAMRMC's major subordinate commands in Figure 2-3. Approximately 4,600 military and civilian personnel are assigned to headquarters and the 12 subordinate units (USAMRMC, 2001a).

As the army's medical materiel developer and logistician, USAMRMC has specified five major core capabilities (USAMRMC, 2001c):

- Medical research and development
- Logistics and acquisition
- Information management/information technology
- Advanced technologies
- Congressional programs

As part of its medical research and development charge, USAMRMC has the responsibility for managing research as well as product development related to, among other things, vaccines and therapeutic agents aimed at preventing and controlling naturally occurring infectious diseases that are perceived to threaten the operational effectiveness of the armed forces. However, USAMRMC does not manage the advanced development of vaccines against biological agents that may be weaponized; DoD assigns that mission to the Joint Vaccine Acquisition Program (JVAP) (see also footnote 13).

Despite its role in vaccine acquisition, USAMRMC is not formally involved in determining DoD policy for vaccine use. The Office of the Assistant Secretary of Defense for Health Affairs (ASD[HA]) is charged with establishing and implementing policies relating to health care services for members of the armed forces. The civilian expert members of the Armed Forces Epidemiological Board (AFEB)—a standing scientific advisory committee under the executive agency of the army established by P.L. 92-463 (AFEB, 2001)—serve as scientific advisers to DoD and address such issues as disease control and health maintenance and disease prevention, including the use of vaccines.

[2]The U.S. Army Garrison at Ft. Detrick is not included in this total, although it is included in Figure 2-3.

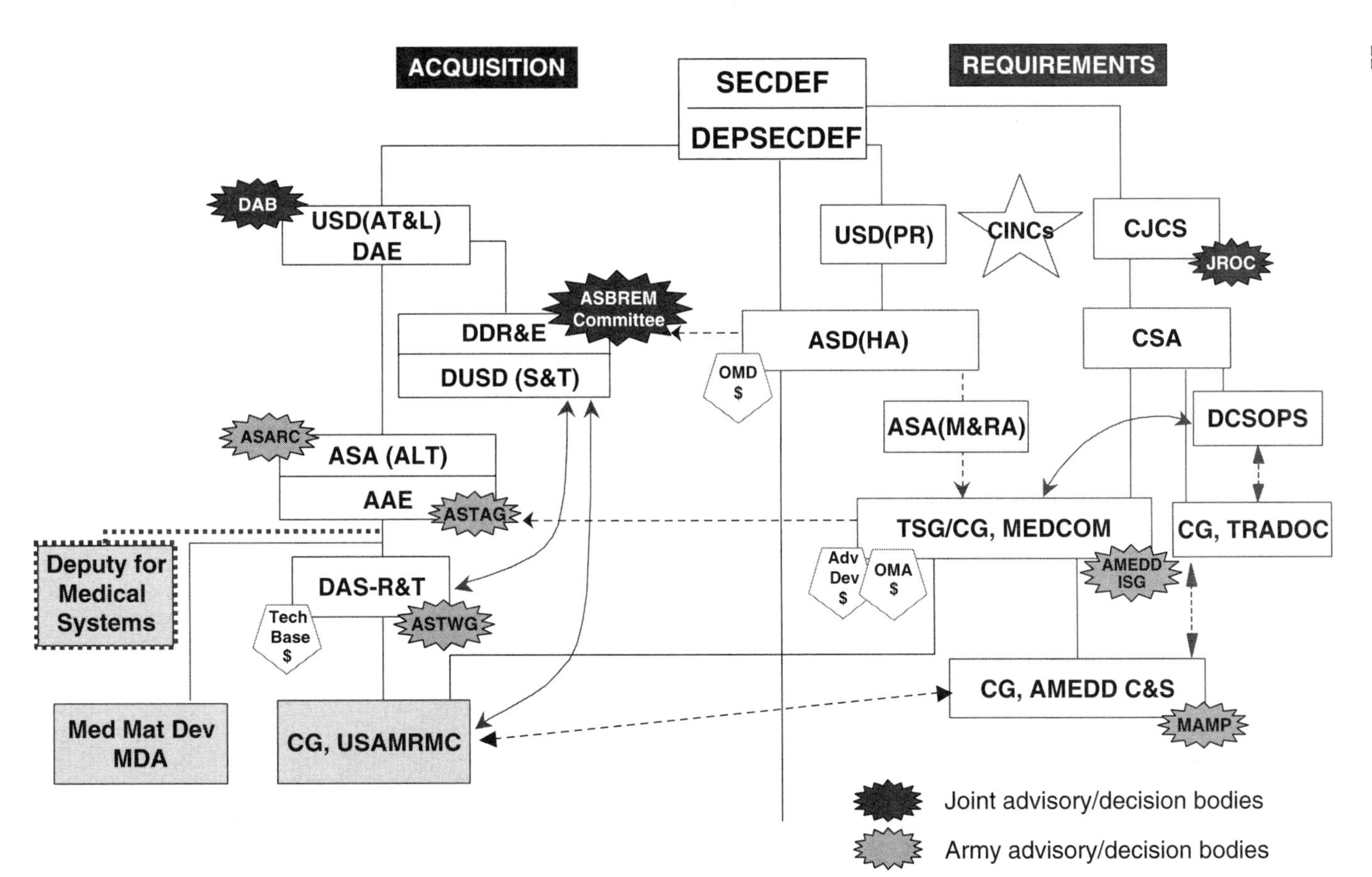

ACQUISITION
SECDEF
DEPSECDEF
REQUIREMENTS
DAB
USD(AT&L)
DAE
USD(PR)
CINCs
CJCS
JROC
ASBREM Committee
DDR&E
DUSD (S&T)
ASD(HA)
OMD $
CSA
ASARC
ASA (ALT)
AAE
ASTAG
ASA(M&RA)
DCSOPS
TSG/CG, MEDCOM
CG, TRADOC
Deputy for Medical Systems
DAS-R&T
Tech Base $
ASTWG
Adv Dev $
OMA $
AMEDD ISG
CG, AMEDD C&S
MAMP
Med Mat Dev MDA
CG, USAMRMC
Joint advisory/decision bodies
Army advisory/decision bodies

FIGURE 2-1 Military infectious disease-related research, development, and acquisition activities: USAMRMC interfaces with army and Office of the Secretary of Defense organizations. Abbreviations: **AAE,** Army Acquisition Executive; **Adv Dev,** advanced development; **AMEDD C&S,** Army Medical Department Center and School; **AMEDD ISG,** Army Medical Department Integration Steering Group; **ASA(ALT),** Assistant Secretary of the Army for Acquisition, Logistics, and Technology; **ASA(M&RA),** Assistant Secretary of the Army for Manpower and Reserve Affairs; **ASBREM,** Armed Services Biomedical Research, Evaluation and Management (Committee); **ASD(HA),** Assistant Secretary of Defense for Health Affairs; **ASARC,** Army Systems Acquisition Review Council; **ASTAG,** Army Science and Technology Advisory Group; **ASTWG,** Army Science and Technology Working Group; **CG,** Commanding General; **CINCs,** Commanders in Chief; **CJCS,** Chairman, Joint Chiefs of Staff; **CSA,** Chief of Staff, U.S. Army; **DAB,** Defense Acquisition Board; **DAE,** Defense Acquisition Executive; **DAS-R&T,** Deputy Assistant Secretary of the Army for Research and Technology; **DCSOPS,** Deputy Chief of Staff for Operations and Plans, U.S. Army; **DDR&E,** Director of Defense Research and Engineering; **DEPSECDEF,** Deputy Secretary of Defense; **DUSD(S&T),** Deputy Under Secretary of Defense for Science and Technology; **JROC,** Joint Requirements Oversight Council; **MAMP,** Mission Area Materiel Plan; **MEDCOM,** Medical Command, U.S. Army; **Med Mat Dev,** medical materiel developer; **OMA,** Operations and Maintenance, U.S. Army; **OMD,** Operations and Maintenance, Department of Defense; **SECDEF,** Secretary of Defense; **Tech Base,** technology base; **TRADOC,** Training and Doctrine Command, U.S. Army; **TSG,** The Surgeon General; **USD(AT&L),** Under Secretary of Defense for Acquisition, Technology, and Logistics; **USAMRMC,** U.S. Army Medical Research and Materiel Command; **USD(PR),** Under Secretary of Defense for Personnel and Readiness. SOURCE: Glenn (2000).

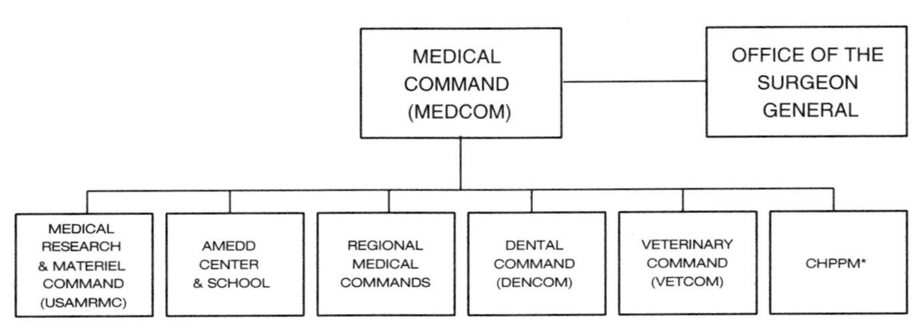

FIGURE 2-2 U.S. Army Medical Department (AMEDD) organizational chart. SOURCE: USAMRMC (2002b).

Basic Research Resources

Medical research and development activities within USAMRMC are conducted at six major laboratories, three laboratory detachments, and three overseas laboratories (USAMRMC, 2001b):

1. U.S. Army Aeromedical Research Laboratory
2. U.S. Army Institute of Surgical Research
3. U.S. Army Medical Research Institute of Chemical Defense
4. U.S. Army Medical Research Institute of Infectious Diseases
5. U.S. Army Research Institute of Environmental Medicine
   - U.S. Army Center for Environmental Health Research
6. Walter Reed Army Institute of Research
   - U.S. Army Dental Research Detachment
   - U.S. Army Medical Research Detachment
   - Armed Forces Research Institute of Medical Sciences—Thailand
   - U.S. Army Medical Research Unit—Europe
   - U.S. Army Medical Research Unit—Kenya

Infectious disease-related research activities are carried out within several of these laboratories, specifically, the Walter Reed Army Institute of Research (WRAIR) in Silver Spring, Maryland; WRAIR's affiliated overseas laboratories

U.S. Army Medical Research and Materiel Command

Commanding General

Office of the Commander and Headquarters Staff

Administrative Support

- Deputy Commander
  - International Activities
- Chief of Staff
  - DCoS, Resource Mgmt
  - DCoS, Operations
  - DCoS, Info Mgmt
  - DCoS, Logistics
  - DCoS, Personnel
- Secretary of the General's Staff
  - Public Affairs Office
  - Protocol Office
- Command Sergeant Major
- Special Staff (PARC, JAG, IR)
- ASA(ALT) Liaison
- Liaison to AMEDD C&S
- Personnel Demonstration Project
- Biological Arms Control Treaty Office (BACTO)

Research Management

- Deputy for Medical Research
  - Director, Research Plans and Programs
  - Research Area Director for Infectious Diseases
  - Research Area Director for Combat Casualty Care
  - Research Area Director for Military Operational Medicine
  - Research Area Director for Chem /Bio Defense
- Deputy for Regulatory Compliance & Quality
- Deputy for Advanced Technology
  - Director, Telemedicine and Advanced Technologies Research Center (TATRC)
- Director for Congressionally Directed Medical Research Programs (CDMRP)

Materiel Development and Acquisition

- Deputy for Acquisition and Advanced Development
- Deputy for Materiel
- Deputy for IM/IT

Major Subordinate Commands

Research Laboratories

- US Army Medical Research Institute of Infectious Diseases (USAMRIID)
- US Army Medical Research Institute of Chemical Defense (USAMRICD)
- US Army Research Institute of Environmental Medicine (USARIEM)
- US Army Center for Environmental Health Research (USACEHR)
- US Army Aeromedical Research Laboratory (USAARL)
- US Army Institute of Surgical Research (USAISR)
- Walter Reed Army Institute of Research (WRAIR)
- US Army Dental Research Detachment (USADRD)
- US Army Medical Research Detachment (USAMRD)
- Armed Forces Research Institute of Medical Sciences (AFRIMS)
- US Army Medical Research Unit Kenya (USAMRU-K)
- US Army Medical Research Unit Europe (USAMRU-E)

Other Commands/Directorates

- US Army Medical Materiel Development Activity (USAMMDA)
- US Army Medical Materiel Agency (USAMMA)
- US Army Medical Materiel Center Europe (USAMMCE)
- US Army Medical Research Acquisition Activity (USAMRAA)
- US Army Health Facilities Planning Agency (HFPA)
- US Army Medical Information Systems & Services Agency (USAMISSA)
- US Army Garrison, Ft. Detrick (USAG) and Site R

FIGURE 2-3 U.S. Army Medical Research and Materiel Command organizational chart. SOURCE: USAMRMC (2001d).

(listed above); and the U.S. Army Medical Research Institute of Infectious Diseases (USAMRIID) at Fort Detrick, Maryland. USAMRIID maintains Biological Safety Level 4 research facilities. This capability permits research to be conducted with lethal pathogens (e.g., viruses that cause hemorrhagic fevers). The WRAIR complex includes a facility for the production of pilot lots of vaccines, which allows scientists to move prototype vaccines rapidly into production under good manufacturing practices (GMP)[3] "that assure [the] purity, quality & consistency" of the product (Goldenthal, 2000).

The military also carries out infectious disease-related research at laboratories operated by the Navy Bureau of Medicine, including those at the Naval Medical Research Center, now colocated with WRAIR, and its affiliated overseas laboratories—the Navy Medical Research Unit 3 in Egypt, the Navy Medical Research Unit 2 (NAMRU-2) in Indonesia, and the Naval Medical Research Center Detachment in Peru.

Military Infectious Diseases Research Program

USAMRMC's core medical research and development program is divided into four research area directorates (RADs) (USAMRMC, 2001a):

- RAD1: Military Infectious Diseases Research Program (MIDRP)
- RAD2: Combat Casualty Care Research Program
- RAD3: Military Operational Medicine Research Program
- RAD4: Medical Chemical and Biological Defense Program

RAD1 is the research directorate that manages MIDRP, which is charged with development of products to protect deployed warfighters against naturally occurring infectious diseases. MIDRP management (represented as Research Area Director for Infectious Diseases in Figure 2-2) coordinates the diverse and diffuse infectious disease-related research and development activities of USAMRMC and, on the basis of congressional direction,[4] coordinates the infectious disease-related research activities of DoD research laboratories worldwide, including laboratories that are not within USAMRMC's direct command, such as the Navy laboratories.

MIDRP's mission is "to conduct, for the Department of Defense, a focused and responsive world class infectious diseases research and development program leading to fielding of effective and improved means of protection and treatment

[3]Current good manufacturing practice in manufacturing, processing, packing, or holding drugs, general. 21 C.F.R. § 210 (2001); Current good manufacturing practice for finished pharmaceuticals. 21 C.F.R. § 211 (2001); Biological Products. 21 C.F.R. § 600 (2001).

[4]Department of Defense Appropriations Act, 1982. P.L. 97-114 (1981).

to maintain maximal global operational capability with minimal morbidity" (Hoke, 2000a, p. 5). USAMRMC cites as support for this program a September 1999 executive order that refers specifically to "diseases endemic to an area of operations" and states that "it is the Policy of the United States Government to provide our military personnel with safe and effective vaccines, antidotes, and treatments that will negate or minimize the effects of these health threats" (Clinton, 1999).

Because it represents the naturally occurring infectious disease-related research interests of USAMRMC, MIDRP's scope could extend to any naturally occurring infectious disease, endemic or newly emerging, that is judged to be capable of influencing the outcome of military operations by producing excessive morbidity, mortality, or disturbances to morale or whose occurrence could result in the excessive consumption of resources. MIDRP operates as a source of information and proponency for vaccine-related research and makes recommendations to the commanding general of USAMRMC regarding the allocation of funds to the organizations that will conduct that research. Approximately 1,000 people—including uniformed and civilian scientists—are available to support the infectious disease-related research mission of USAMRMC (Hoke, 2000a).

A summary of fiscal year (FY) 2002 USAMRMC infectious disease-related research funding is shown in Table 2-1.

TABLE 2-1 USAMRMC Infectious Disease-Related Research Funding,[a] FY 2002 (in millions)

Budget Activity[b]	Vaccine	Other	Total
6.1 Basic research	2.8	6.5	9.3
6.2 Exploratory development	20.7	11.6	32.3
6.3 Advanced development	7.9	6.3	14.2
MIDRP funding total	31.4	24.4	55.8
6.4 Demonstration and validation	3.8	0.2	4.0
6.5 Engineering and manufacturing development	2.1	1.2	3.3
Advanced development funding total	5.9	1.4	7.3

[a]The MIDRP director explained that figures given include relevant funding for the Science and Technology Evaluation Program and Science and Technology Objectives. WRAIR overhead is a large item that is distributed in proportion to the size of the two types of support. The figures in this table do not include human immunodeficiency virus-related research activities, which are included on a separate funding line.

[b]Decisions related to the allocation of 6.1 to 6.3 funds rest with MIDRP; decisions related to the allocation of 6.4 and 6.5 funds do not.

SOURCE: Hoke (2002).

Advanced Development and Logistics Resources

Intersecting with the basic laboratory-based research and development activities that MIDRP coordinates are USAMRMC's advanced development and logistics management functions (Major Subordinate Commands listed in Figure 2-3), which include the following (USAMRMC, 2001a):

- Advanced development:
  U.S. Army Medical Materiel Development Agency (USAMMDA)
- Contracting:
  U.S. Army Medical Research Acquisition Activity (USAMRAA)
- Medical logistics:
  U.S. Army Medical Materiel Activity (USAMMA) and
  U.S. Army Medical Materiel Center Europe
- Health facilities planning:
  Health Facilities Planning Agency

Three of the four major subordinate commands of USAMRMC play significant roles in the vaccine acquisition process: USAMMDA, USAMRAA, and USAMMA. The USAMRMC website describes the responsibilities of these subordinate commands as follows (USAMRMC, 2001a, p. 23):

> The U.S. Army Medical Materiel Development Activity (USAMMDA), Fort Detrick, Maryland, develops and fields medical products for U.S. Armed Forces, in conjunction with the Army Medical Department Center and School (the medical combat developer) and the U.S. Army Medical Materiel Activity (the medical logistician). Concepts/products developed in the USAMRMC laboratories are transitioned to USAMMDA for advanced development. USAMMDA plans, manages, and directs execution of medical materiel development to achieve U.S. Army and Joint Service materiel system objectives to meet cost, schedule, and performance. The USAMMDA also manages clinical data and coordinates with the Food and Drug Administration for approval of medical materiel for human use. The USAMMDA's vision is to provide world-class medical solutions for U.S. warfighters.
>
> The U.S. Army Medical Research Acquisition Activity (USAMRAA), Fort Detrick, Maryland, provides contracting support to the USAMRMC and its worldwide network of laboratories, to the Fort Detrick Army Garrison, military tenant activities, Army-wide projects sponsored by The Surgeon General, and congressionally mandated programs. The USAMRAA vision is to be a leader in innovation and the premier federal organization committed to acquisition excellence. The USAMRAA staff has leaders in innovation who are committed to acquisition excellence. They provide expert advice on procurement and assistance issues.
>
> The U.S. Army Medical Materiel Agency (USAMMA), Fort Detrick, Maryland, serves as the Army Surgeon General's central focal point and executive agent for all strategic medical logistics. Its mission is to deliver and sustain responsive medical logistics support for all worldwide military health care operations. The USAMMA serves as the AMEDD's [Army Medical Department] fielding command for all new medical materiel, and centrally manages a variety of strategic logistics programs such as war reserve and critical item asset management, deployment of materiel handoff teams, and operational oversight of medical materiel acquisition vehicles. Core skills and technologies center on conducting

life-cycle management for commercial and nondevelopmental items, sustaining and modernizing the medical force, supporting exercises and contingency operations, and promoting medical logistics information and knowledge. USAMMA personnel develop and implement innovative logistics concepts and technologies, manage strategic war reserve and critical items (e.g., anthrax vaccine), and manage the acquisition life cycle for medical materiel.

RESEARCH, DEVELOPMENT, AND ACQUISITION IN CONTEXT

To make the journey from a recognized military medical problem to a licensed and procured or available vaccine, an idea must pass through a complex series of priority-setting and budgeting processes and through the hands of various USAMRMC managers, as well as numerous DoD stakeholders outside USAMRMC. Research priorities evolve through multiple channels. Officially, a military product begins life as a perceived need—a problem that needs a solution. Needs are first formalized as Future Operational Capabilities (FOCs). FOCs are worded very generally and allow consideration of solutions based on doctrine,[5] training, leader development, organization, materiel (products), or the soldier (DA, 1999). Preference is given to the quickest, least expensive solutions (often those that involve doctrine) over the slowest, most expensive solutions (often those that involve materiel) (DA, 1999).

MIDRP, with input from the service requirements offices, drafts product-related objectives for review and modification by the Joint Technology Coordinating Group-2,[6] recommends draft objectives to the USAMRMC commanding general, and develops research plans that reflect the goals outlined in FOCs.

Regarding materiel solutions for infectious diseases, FOCs allow, for instance, consideration of vaccines, drugs, immunotherapies, immunoprophylactic preparations, vector control products, and diagnostic tests. As part of its threat identification and prioritization duties, the Army Medical Department (AMEDD) Center and School[7] reviews the products that are being sought through MIDRP and offers an assessment of their importance, providing feedback to MIDRP about its priorities. Informal dialogue between MIDRP and the AMEDD Center and School is ongoing, and inputs on infectious diseases threats are obtained from a number

[5]Doctrine is defined as "fundamental principles by which the military forces or elements thereof guide their actions in support of national objections. It is authoritative but requires judgment in application" (DTIC, 2002).

[6]According to the recommendations of AFEB, the Joint Technology Coordinating Group-2, a subunit of the Armed Services Biomedical Research Evaluation and Management (ASBREM) system, includes representatives from each service and seeks to coordinate infectious disease-related research among the services (AFEB, 1991).

[7]The AMEDD Center and School's Directorate of Combat and Doctrine Development establishes concepts, requirements, doctrine, organizational structure, and equipment needs for all medical functions of the Army (Scott, 2000). Other DoD commands similarly address these tasks through command centers and schools.

of sources.[8] The AMEDD Center and School also has the responsibility to produce a list of infectious disease threats (Scott, 2000). However, the most recent threat list produced by AMEDD Center and School (approved by U.S. Army Training and Doctrine Command [TRADOC]) was produced in 1986, with modifications in 1987 and 1988 (Hoke, 2002; TRADOC, 1986).

The Assistant Secretary of the Army for Acquisition, Logistics, and Technology (ASA[ALT]) provides funds to support technology base-related research efforts (6.1 through 6.3 research). MIDRP provides guidance regarding research priority setting and manages the distribution of funds for that research (Table 2-1). Each year, army research and development laboratories—both medical and nonmedical—submit to ASA(ALT) nominations of products to be selected as Army Science and Technology Objectives (STOs). STOs are identified, refined, reviewed, and prioritized annually through a process that involves input from a large number of interested parties, including USAMRMC,[9] leading to final approval of the STO program by TRADOC.[10] Approved STOs receive priority funding (TRADOC, 1999). Multiyear funding for research is not available without a STO. Within USAMRMC, the promise to provide specified STO funding is considered firm. At present there are about 200 STOs throughout the army. Of those, approximately 30 STOs are medical, and 8 of those[11] are within the purview of MIDRP.

---

[8]The Armed Forces Medical Intelligence Center, part of the Defense Intelligence Agency, maintains current knowledge of foreign medical and technology capabilities, environmental risks, and infectious disease epidemiology to produce geographically focused assessments of threats. Resources within DoD also contribute indirectly to the identification and prioritization of the need for vaccines against infectious diseases. For instance, a number of DoD units gather information, such as the U.S. Army Center for Health Promotion and Preventive Medicine, which operates the Army Medical Surveillance Activity. Navy and air force units, such as the Naval Health Research Center's Center for Deployment Health Research and the Force Health Protection and Surveillance Branch at Brooks Air Force Base, collect international information relating to epidemiology, disease surveillance, and biological research. The DoD Global Emerging Infections Surveillance and Response System, for which the army is the lead agent, also contributes to global infectious disease surveillance and response efforts. It is the committee's understanding that these inputs theoretically enter into the infectious disease threat assessment and prioritization process through the AMEDD Center and School. Sources outside the DoD (e.g., the National Intelligence Council) also gather valuable infectious disease surveillance-related information.

[9]MIDRP formulates objectives and presents them to a Joint Working Group (JWG) for comment. JWG is in a state of evolution. The commanders of the laboratories (WRAIR, USAMRIID, and Naval Medical Research Center), their scientific directors, the members of the Joint Technology Coordinating Group-2, and the USAMRMC Deputy for Research and Development are on the JWG (Hoke, 2002).

[10]In a separate process, the Armed Services Biomedical Research Evaluation and Management Committee (ASBREM) requests nominations of products as Defense Technology Objectives (DTOs). ASBREM, which provides joint oversight of and focus for DoD biomedical science and technology (Glenn, 2000), designates medical DTOs and monitors their progress through an annual Technology Area Review and Assessment.

[11]Current vaccine-related STO areas include a multiantigen, multistage *Plasmodium vivax* malaria vaccine; a multistage, multiantigen recombinant *Plasmodium falciparum* malaria vaccine; prevention

New product development efforts may begin without formal documentation of a specific need. In addition to formal STO efforts, USAMRMC maintains other basic research activities under its Science and Technology Evaluation Program (STEP). When enough is known to allow formulation of a specific product plan, USAMRMC can then propose it as a STO.

In FY 2001, infectious disease vaccine-related research[12] STEPs included work on malaria vaccines, means for the prevention of diarrheal diseases, flavivirus vaccines, the malaria genome project, hepatitis virus vaccines, meningococcal vaccines, vaccine delivery, protection from viruses that cause hemorrhagic fevers and other highly lethal viruses, rickettsial diseases, and the prevention of human immunodeficiency virus (HIV) infections in military personnel (Hoke, 2000a). Figure 2-4 outlines the research and development path for vaccines.

At the end of the 6.3 program phase, projects are reviewed to determine their suitability for advanced development. If a successful candidate (in the context of this report, a candidate vaccine against a naturally occurring infectious disease) emerges from the research and development technology base—the domain of MIDRP—it is transitioned to the advanced development stage, at which time the product leaves MIDRP management and becomes the charge of USAMMDA,[13] another part of USAMRMC. The transition to advanced development requires formal documentation—in the form of an Operational Requirements Document (ORD)—of a specific need for the product. An ORD specifies performance and other operational parameters for the product, including estimates of the funds that will be required, personnel requirements, and measurable capabilities and characteristics of the proposed system (DoD, 2001e). Typically, 5 to 10 years might pass after the start of work on a product before an ORD is written.

Once MIDRP recommends a product for transition to advanced development, a USAMMDA product manager works with a research coordinator to collect information and prepare a development plan. The vaccine product is then presented to representatives of other DoD organizational elements involved in the acquisition and procurement of medical materiel for approval. The core team members are the combat developer (AMEDD Center and School), the materiel developer (USAMMDA), and the logistician (USAMMA). Whether the potential product makes the transition to advanced development depends on an assessment

---

of diarrheal diseases; and nucleic acid (DNA)-based vaccines to prevent dengue (ASA[ALT], 2001; Hoke, 2002).

[12]These are therefore within MIDRP's charge.

[13]Candidate vaccines for use against biological agents that may be weaponized are instead transitioned to the Joint Vaccine Acquisition Program, JVAP. The Joint Vaccine Acquisition Program, begun in 1996 as an outgrowth of a 1994 law directing DoD to coordinate its biodefense activities (National Defense Authorization Act for Fiscal Year 1994, P.L. 103-60 [1993]; Johnson-Winegar, 2000), is charged with coordinating the acquisition process for vaccines and other medical products effective against validated biological warfare threat agents (JVAP, 2001).

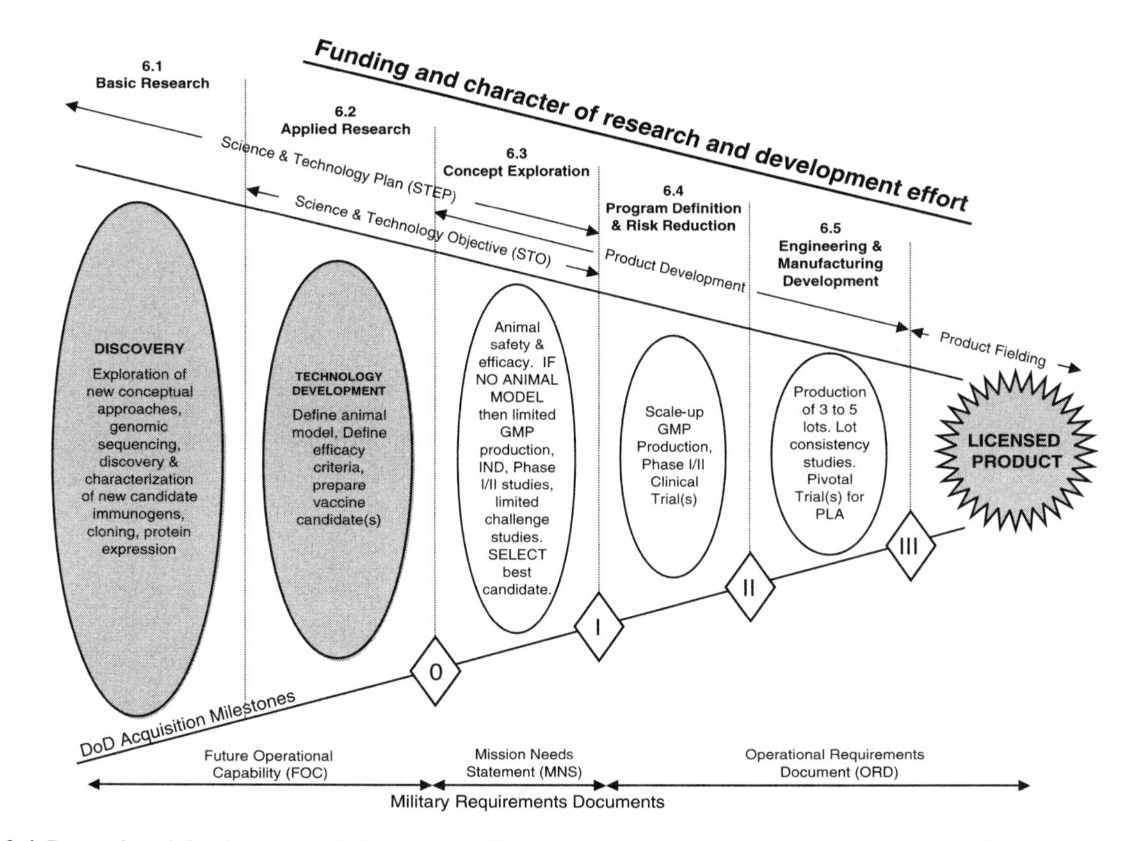

FIGURE 2-4 Research and development path for vaccines. The army changed the "milestone" nomenclature depicted in this figure after its presentation to this committee. The general flow of activity is, however, correctly shown. SOURCE: Hoke (2000b).

of technical feasibility, need, and the availability of funds. At this point in the process, products are categorized on the basis of the estimated total program cost (DoD, 2001e). Acquisition categories (ACATs) determine the level of DoD review, decision authority, and the procedures applicable for a given acquisition project (DoD, 2001e). At present, each vaccine product is managed as a distinct acquisition system. Vaccine products are managed as ACAT III (less than major) systems, the lowest priority of the three ACAT levels (i.e., ACAT I, ACAT II, and ACAT III) (DoD, 2002; Personal communication, W. Howell, Department of Defense, February 28, 2002).[14]

Consideration has been (and continues to be) given to packaging vaccines together in project groups to increase their visibility within DoD and, subsequently, to increase their opportunities for funding. Also, a planned reorganization of the advanced development is to be implemented in July 2002.[15] This reorganization is intended to refine the management of acquisition activities within USAMRMC. Cumulatively, these changes are to bring USAMRMC acquisition practices more in line with DoD norms. These changes will not, however, directly affect basic research and development (vis-à-vis MIDRP).

The vaccine product competes with other products for funding for advanced development and other resources, such as staff expertise. The funding path for advanced development research (6.4 and 6.5) originates with the Deputy Chief of Staff for Operations and Plans, U.S. Army (DCSOPS) and differs from the funding path for technology base research (6.1 through 6.3). Funding for advanced development of vaccines against infectious diseases is substantially less (approximately $7.3 million total in FY 2002) than funding for technology base research funding ($55.8 million total in FY 2002; see also Table 2-1). At present approximately seven[16] (Hoke, 2002) vaccine products are in advanced development.

Progress to advanced development can stall even though a technically feasible product candidate may have been worked on for years. For instance, limited

---

[14]The highest-priority systems, ACAT I systems, are those systems estimated by the Under Secretary of Defense for Acquisition, Technology, and Logistics (USD[AT&L]) to require an eventual total expenditure for research, development, testing, and evaluation of more than $365 million (in constant FY 2000 dollars) or an eventual total expenditure for procurement of more than $2.19 billion. ACAT II and ACAT III programs are both considered nonmajor defense acquisition programs, although the oversight mechanisms differ between them (DoD, 2001e).

[15]According to USAMRMC staff, the planned reorganization will form four advanced development project areas: (1) information technology management, (2) pharmaceutical development, (3) devices development, and (4) commercial off-the-shelf nondevelopment. Each project area will have a project manager. Each project manager may in turn be responsible for a number of product managers (e.g., all malaria-related products [drugs, vaccines, etc.] will have one product manager) (Personal communication, W. Howell, Department of Defense, March 5, 2002).

[16]Including a wholecell, recombinant subunit vaccine against enterotoxigenic *Escherichia coli*, a vaccine against *Campylobacter*, a vaccine against *Shigella flexneri* type 2A (SC602), a recombinant vaccine against malaria (RTS,S), tetravalent vaccines against dengue, hepatitis E vaccines, and HIV vaccines (Hoke, 2002).

funds may be directed to projects that DoD considers—according to official priority ranking or by decision-maker discretion—to be relatively more important. Diseases may be sufficiently localized or so rare that populations appropriate for efficacy testing are not available; or projects may face financial, ethical, or regulatory constraints. Also, in the absence of partners in advanced development of a product, further basic scientific development may be impractical.

Successful advanced development efforts proceed from advanced clinical trials and upscaling of manufacturing for Phase III efficacy trials through to the submission of a Biologics License Application to the Food and Drug Administration.

PROCUREMENT, STORAGE, AND DISTRIBUTION IN CONTEXT

Within DoD, funds for the purchase of medical products and the maintenance of medical products that have been acquired (including vaccines) are separate from funds for research and development. Program 6 funds are used to fund 6.1 through 6.5 research and development, and Program 8 funds are used to fund operations and maintenance.

Once a product is licensed, AFEB and other organizations consider recommendations for use of the product by military personnel. Each service is responsible for procuring its own required vaccines in coordination with USAMMA, the designated lead agent for vaccine supply (AFEB, 1999). Medical care facilities purchase vaccine products recommended for routine use for the protection of the health of the members of the armed forces (e.g., adenovirus vaccine), usually directly from the vendor. Vaccine products recommended for use for the protection of new recruits or for general use among all members of the armed services are procured with funds for medical care (Defense Health Care). The USAMRMC commanding general has no authority in this process. Some vaccines recommended for use in specific deployments do, however, fall within the nominal authority of USAMRMC through USAMMA.

Vaccines that are DoD-wide requirements may be purchased from stocks held by the Defense Logistics Agency and its inventory control point, the Defense Supply Center, Philadelphia (DSCP). At the time of this writing, DSCP reports that it stocks influenza and yellow fever vaccines (Hoke, 2002). Vaccines of importance to the military that DSCP does not stock include those that are no longer available (those for the prevention of adenovirus infection, cholera, Lyme disease, and plague) as well as those otherwise available to prevent *Haemophilus influenzae* type B infection; hepatitis A; hepatitis B; Japanese encephalitis; measles, mumps, and rubella; meningococcal disease; pneumococcal disease; polio (the inactivated vaccine); rabies; tetanus; diphtheria; typhoid; and varicella (DSCP, 2002). DSCP manages the procurement and distribution only of those vaccines that are licensed by the Food and Drug Administration (AFEB, 1999). Available vaccines that DSCP does not stock are usually obtained directly from the manufacturer on an as-needed basis. Some purchase agreements (prime vendor agreements) include clauses that obligate a supplier to meet military needs during surges in demand (DMM, 2002). However, shortages and other supply issues can affect timely access to many of the vaccines listed above that are otherwise considered putatively available (DSCP, 2002).

EXTERNAL INTERACTIONS

A number of cooperative agreements facilitate DoD's research efforts, including Collaborative Research and Development Agreements (CRADAs), Small Business Innovation Research awards, Dual-Use Science and Technology (DUST) agreements, and other mechanisms. DoD uses these agreements to secure relationships with companies, academic institutions, the governments of other nations, and U.S. government agencies other than DoD.[17] USAMRAA processes and monitors internal and external agreements.

The CRADA is a common mechanism used to make external vaccine-related research and development agreements and one of the few means by which DoD can accept resources from external sources. In late 2001, as many as 78 infectious disease-related CRADAs involving as many as 69 partners were active (Hoke, 2002). Laboratory commanders or USAMRMC negotiate CRADAs. Partners use CRADAs to form collaborative relationships, often for the development of specific products. CRADAs allow DoD's partners to supply DoD with people and in-kind resources. Laboratory commanders use CRADAs to acquire additional resources to work on products that are related to the objectives of MIDRP, extending their work into research areas where limited resources do not permit full government funding (Booz Allen and Hamilton, 1999, p. 17). As a result DoD laboratories may incur obligations to partner companies. Despite its charge to oversee research related to infectious diseases, the MIDRP management office (RAD1) reports that it is neither involved in CRADA development or approval nor routinely informed of the terms of such arrangements.

The DUST program supports initiatives that may have some use in the civilian sector as well as utility to the military. The program is funded by DoD dollars drawn from research and development funds. A complex formula governs the amounts provided by companies and by the government. Scientists initiate DUST agreements to take advantage of the available funds. In contrast to the approval process for CRADAs, the MIDRP management office reports that it is heavily involved in the review of proposed DUST agreements, providing input regarding feasibility and program relevance.

Examples of current partnerships are shown in Table 2-2.

---

[17]Some agreements are wholly internal to DoD, such as when USAMMDA enters into agreements with DoD medical research laboratories (e.g., USAMRIID or overseas medical research laboratories) for advanced development of products that emerged from the DoD technology research base.

TABLE 2-2 Selected Current Vaccine-Related Agreements

Award Type	Partner Organization	Project Title
DUST agreement		
	Acambis, Inc.	Development of a live attenuated vaccine for the prevention of diarrhea caused by enterotoxigenic *Escherichia coli* (ETEC)
	Acambis, Inc.	Development of a subunit vaccine for the prevention of *Campylobacter* infection
Small Business Innovation Research		
	3rd Millennium Inc.	Development of World Wide Web-driven bioinformatic platform of DNA microarrays
	Eikos LLC	Platforms for rapid DNA microarray prototyping
Small Business Technology Transfer		
	Antex Biologics Inc.	Development of a prototype multivalent oral vaccine for travelers
CRADA		
	Multiple partners include: • U.S. government agencies • Non-U.S. government agencies • Pharmaceutical companies • Biotechnology companies • U.S. academic institutions • Non-U.S. academic institutions	Examples of projects include: • Research of candidate vaccines for the prevention of HIV infection and AIDS • Development of a cholera vaccine for military personnel • Research and development of vaccine products against ETEC • Malaria vaccine development • Shigella vaccine development

SOURCE: Adapted from Hoke (2002).

Government Agencies and Nongovernment Organizations

Many international organizations and U.S. agencies other than DoD share USAMRMC's vaccine development mission to various degrees, although their resources, specific areas of focus, and underlying purposes and the populations that they serve may differ. From MIDRP's perspective, the National Institutes of Health (NIH) is a critical contributor to basic infectious disease-related research.

NIH recently opened the Vaccine Research Center. NIH has devoted substantial funds to globally important infectious disease-related research, and some of this research is also of interest to USAMRMC (such as research on HIV—$2.8 billion/year [NIH, 2002b]—and malaria—$71 million/year [Personal communication, W. Crum, NIAID Office of Financial Management, June 14, 2002]). A dramatic increase in NIH funding for research on biological agents that may be weaponized, totaling $1.5 billion for the National Institute of Allergy and Infectious Diseases alone, is requested in the President's proposed FY 2003 budget (NIH, 2002a).

The Centers for Disease Control and Prevention (CDC) conducts outbreak investigations and disease control efforts and has been charged with, for example, the creation of a new national stockpile of smallpox vaccine (Gordon, 2001). CDC also maintains stockpiles of vaccines—mostly mandated pediatric vaccines such as the measles-mumps-rubella vaccine, tetanus-diphtheria toxoid, and inactivated polio vaccine—through the companies that manufacture the vaccines to ensure continued access to these vaccines for public health. CDC is considering whether to stock new vaccines, such as Wyeth's pneumococcal conjugate vaccine, Prevnar, and Merck's varicella vaccine, Varivax (Vaccine Stockpile Strategy, 2002). Although the Food and Drug Administration's role is mostly regulatory, the agency also maintains a research capability in biologics evaluation and research and contributes to DoD's research programs through the CRADA mechanism.

International organizations such as the World Health Organization and its regional affiliates (such as the Pan American Health Organization) also undertake vaccine-related research and development and facilitate the development of programs to control vaccine-preventable diseases. Many DoD medical research laboratories serve as reference laboratories for CDC (e.g., USAMRIID) (USAMRMC, 2001a) and the World Health Organization (e.g., NAMRU-2) (NAMRU-2, undated).

Interactions among these organizations and between these organizations and DoD vary in their levels of formality, extent, and effectiveness. At present, some program-level coordination of research efforts between DoD and other federal agencies and international organizations exists. DoD representatives participate in the National Vaccine Program Office Interagency Group, and DoD sends liaisons to the National Vaccine Advisory Committee (NVPO, 2001). The DoD research program in retrovirology is in frequent contact with HIV vaccine development offices at NIH. DoD, NIH, and CDC voluntarily coordinate their malaria vaccine programs through the Federal Malaria Vaccine Coordinating Committee (FMVCC, 2001).

Academia

DoD also maintains relationships with academic researchers and institutions for vaccine-related research and development. These relationships exist primarily at the research laboratory level. For example, NIH provides funds to the University of Massachusetts at Worcester to study the pathogenesis of dengue hemorrhagic fever. The bulk of the field research funded through this grant is carried out at the Armed Forces Research Institute of Medical Sciences, a subsidiary of WRAIR, and at other institutions in Thailand. MIDRP also provides funding for these projects. Although this collaboration is not specifically vaccine related, MIDRP considers it to be productive because it lays substantial groundwork that will be needed to field-test an anticipated vaccine against dengue virus.

MIDRP seeks input from academia through its peer review program for proposed research. Since 1999, all internal research funded by MIDRP at army and navy laboratories has been subject to review by external scientists.

Industry

DoD's relationships with industry are complex. USAMRMC research laboratories interact with industry at the vaccine research and development stage (see Table 2-2 for examples) and at the vaccine procurement stage. Successful partnerships have been developed for the procurement of vaccines against influenza virus, Japanese encephalitis virus, and hepatitis A virus. Difficulties with procurement and maintenance have, however, halted or threatened the continued production of vaccines that are needed, such as vaccines against adenovirus, plague, and tetanus (Hoke, 2002). Over the years DoD has developed vaccines against diseases including Rift Valley fever, Argentine hemorrhagic fever, eastern equine encephalitis, western equine encephalitis, and Venezuelan equine encephalitis for which no commercial manufacturers have been identified.

Vaccines developed or marketed by foreign manufacturers for locally endemic diseases may be of use to DoD from time to time (e.g., the vaccine against Japanese encephalitis virus). Other vaccine products (e.g., the vaccine against tick-borne encephalitis) have followed or are following similar development and marketing paths but have not yet been licensed.

Also of note are instances in which a vaccine developed by the Army might have international use that is greater than its direct use to the DoD (e.g., Rift Valley fever). A 1990 analysis suggests that nearly 80 percent of the difference in disease burden between the poorest and richest 20 percent of the world's population, in terms of death and disability-adjusted years, was attributable to communicable disease (Widdus, 2001). Many of the vaccines developed to protect deployed U.S. forces may also be of benefit to the world's poorest populations, perhaps compelling DoD interest in a wider range of vaccine development efforts than might be dictated by market forces alone. The committee observes that, overall, the availability of a vaccine for military use is subject to many complex and changeable interests within—and external to—DoD.

3

Current Status of Vaccines for Military Personnel

The Department of Defense (DoD) administers 17 different vaccines, as outlined in the Joint Instruction on Immunizations and Chemoprophylaxis (Secretaries of the Air Force, Army, Navy, and Transportation, 1995), for the prevention of infectious diseases among military personnel, where appropriate. The vaccines are administered to military personnel on the basis of military occupation, the location of the deployment, and mission requirements. In this chapter, the committee reviews information on the current availability of vaccines to DoD and describes key projects in DoD's vaccine development pipeline.

CURRENT STATUS OF VACCINES FOR MILITARY USE

Table 3-1 provides an overview of the major infectious disease threats to U.S. military personnel and displays whether the appropriate vaccine product is available for military use, is licensed in the United States by the Food and Drug Administration (FDA), is an investigational new drug (IND), or is in development. It is an incomplete list of potential threats and does not include a number of infectious diseases or infectious disease agents for which a vaccine is neither available nor in development, but against which the military might have a need for a vaccine, such as Crimean-Congo hemorrhagic fever, West Nile encephalitis, Nipah virus, Norwalk virus, Lassa fever, and other common infections or infectious disease agents, such as gonorrhea, chlamydia, and tuberculosis. The information presented in the tables that follow are based on material provided by the U.S. Army Medical Research and Materiel Command (USAMRMC), FDA, and the Pharmaceutical Research and Manufacturers of America (PhRMA) websites, as well as presentations made to the committee.

TABLE 3-1 Status of Vaccines for Specific Infectious Disease Threats to the U.S. Military

	Vaccine Available		Vaccine Not Available			
Infectious Disease or Infectious Disease Agent	Licensed by FDA	IND	Licensed by FDA	Had Been Licensed by FDA	Had Been an IND	In Development
Adenovirus types 4 and 7				X		X[a]
Anthrax	X					X[b]
Argentine hemorrhagic fever (Junin virus)		X[c]				
Botulism (botulinum toxin)		X				
Campylobacter						X
Chikungunya fever		X[c]				
Cholera				X		X
Dengue						X
Diphtheria	X					
Eastern equine encephalitis		X[c]				
Ebola virus						X
Enterotoxigenic *Escherichia coli* (ETEC)						X
Hantavirus						X
Hepatitis A	X					
Hepatitis B	X					
Hepatitis C						X
Hepatitis E						X
Human immunodeficiency virus						X
Influenza	X					
Japanese encephalitis	X					X
Leishmaniasis						X
Lyme disease			X			
Malaria						X
Measles	X					
Meningococcal groups A, C, Y, and W-135	X					
Meningococcal group B						X
Mumps	X					
Plague			X			X
Pneumococcal	X					
Poliovirus types I, II, and III	X					
Q fever		X[c]				
Rabies	X					
Rift Valley fever		X[c]				
Rubella	X					
Scrub typhus						X
Shigella						X

continued

TABLE 3-1 Continued

	Vaccine Available		Vaccine Not Available			
Infectious Disease or Infectious Disease Agent	Licensed by FDA	IND	Licensed by FDA	Had Been Licensed by FDA	Had Been an IND	In Development
Smallpox	X[c,d]					X
Tetanus	X					
Tick-borne encephalitis[e]					X	X
Tularemia		X[c]				
Typhoid fever	X					
Varicella	X					
Venezuelan equine encephalitis		X[c]				X
Western equine encephalitis		X[c]				
Yellow fever	X					

[a] DoD awarded Barr Laboratories a contract (September 25, 2001) to develop and manufacture adenovirus type 4 and 7 vaccines (DoD, 2001b).
[b] Several anthrax vaccines are in development, including two by DoD and one by the National Institutes of Health (Johannes and McGinley, 2001).
[c] For special use only; the vaccine has a limited availability and is no longer being produced (Pittman, 2000).
[d] DHHS initially contracted OraVax (now a part of Acambis, Inc.) to produce 50 million doses of a cell culture smallpox vaccine (Acambis, Inc., 2000). After the events of September 11, 2001, and the anthrax mailings in October 2001, the Department of Health and Human Services expanded its contract. The $428 million contract with Acambis, Inc. (and its subcontractor, Baxter International), is to produce 155 million additional doses of the smallpox vaccine (DHHS, 2001). DynPort Vaccine Corporation, DoD's prime vendor contractor through the Joint Vaccine Acquisition Program, has linked with BioReliance to produce 300,000 doses of a smallpox vaccine (Brownlee, 2001; Johnson-Winegar, 2001).
[e] The tick-borne encephalitis vaccine is not licensed or available in the United States but is available in Europe (USAMMDA, 2001a).

SOURCES: Adapted from DoD (2001a), FDA (2001b, 2002a), NIAID (2000), PhRMA (2000), Pittman (2000), USAMRMC (1999), and Zoon and Goldman (2002).

The committee is not aware of a standard definition of the term "vaccine availability" or of any threshold for determining whether a vaccine should be considered available. Some vaccines are available only through difficult and unusual processes or circumstances. For example, special operations troops may be at risk for smallpox, and in such cases arrangements must be made to transfer the smallpox vaccine from the Centers for Disease Control and Prevention (CDC) to DoD.[1] Some vaccines are manufactured in small pilot lots and are available as INDs through DoD's Special Immunizations Program (SIP) to "individuals who have a high occupational risk—laboratory workers, facilities inspectors, vaccine manufacturers and certain military response teams" (Boudreau and Kortepeter, 2002). The precision displayed in Tables 3-1 to 3-5 by the use of dichotomies such as "limited availability" or "unavailable," although helpful as an overview, belies a fluid and complex actuality. At a minimum, the names of the manufacturers keep changing as corporate entities merge, grow, or realign themselves. International coordination is required for some vaccines that are manufactured outside of the United States but licensed in the United States by FDA. Others are manufactured and licensed outside the United States, presenting different and usually more complex acquisition problems.

Nonetheless, the 51 infectious disease threats listed in Tables 3-2 through 3-5 are classified according to the availability of related, specific vaccine products or other biological countermeasures. Specifically, Table 3-2 lists vaccines that are licensed and generally available for use by DoD personnel. It also lists the number of manufacturers involved. Table 3-2 demonstrates that most of these vaccines are manufactured by single suppliers and thereby suggests the fragility of the vaccine supply essential to military readiness. Table 3-3 lists vaccines that were previously licensed by FDA but that are no longer available to DoD. This list includes vaccines against smallpox and plague, further illustrating the armed forces' vulnerability to potential biological warfare agents. Tables 3-4 and 3-5 list vaccines that, although never licensed by FDA, have at times been available for DoD use as products with IND status. Table 3-4 lists those vaccines that are available only under the restrictive regulations governing the use of products with IND status, whereas Table 3-5 lists the subset of products that are no longer produced but that are available to a limited number of military personnel as INDs through DoD's SIP.

Many of the special-use vaccines that were once licensed or used by the military as products with IND status are no longer available. This situation arises as a result of any of a variety of obstacles. For most vaccines that are products with IND status, there was simply insufficient funding for advanced development. For other products, it was deemed difficult, if not impossible, to demonstrate their effectiveness and safety in humans, thus preventing the possibility of their licensure. Market factors, such as inadequate sustained demand, are obstacles as are a lack of interest or monetary incentive for industry to participate in the development or scale-up of the production process, the lack of an adequate physical infrastructure to meet the regulatory requirements for manufacture of the

---

[1]DynPort Vaccine Corporation, DoD's prime vendor contractor through the Joint Vaccine Acquisition Program, has linked with BioReliance to produce a smallpox vaccine. The vaccine is being evaluated at the University of Kentucky, and Phase I clinical trials began in April 2002 (Gay, 2002; Johnson-Winegar, 2001) .

TABLE 3-2 FDA-Licensed Vaccines and Related Biologics Available to U.S. Military Personnel

Product	Manufacturer(s)
Anthrax vaccine, adsorbed	BioPort Corporation
Botulism antitoxin[a]	Aventis Pasteur, Inc.
Hepatitis A vaccine, inactivated	GlaxoSmithKline Biologicals
	Merck & Co., Inc.
Hepatitis A, inactivated, and hepatitis B (recombinant) vaccine	GlaxoSmithKline Biologicals
Hepatitis B vaccine, recombinant	GlaxoSmithKline Biologicals
	Merck & Co., Inc.
Influenza virus vaccine, trivalent, types A and B, current (2001–2002) formula	Aventis Pasteur, Inc.
	Evans Vaccines Limited
	Wyeth Vaccines
Japanese encephalitis virus vaccine, inactivated	Research Foundation for Microbial Diseases of Osaka University (Biken)
Measles virus vaccine, live, attenuated	Merck & Co., Inc.
Measles and mumps virus vaccine, live	Merck & Co., Inc.
Measles, mumps, and rubella virus vaccine, live	Merck & Co., Inc.
Meningococcal polysaccharide vaccine, groups A, C, Y, and W-135	Aventis Pasteur, Inc.
Mumps virus vaccine, live	Merck & Co., Inc.
Pneumococcal 7-valent conjugate vaccine	Wyeth Vaccines
Pneumococcal polysaccharide polyvalent vaccine	Wyeth Vaccines
	Merck & Co., Inc.
Poliovirus vaccine, inactivated	Aventis Pasteur, SA
Rabies immune globulin	Aventis Pasteur, SA
	Bayer Corporation
Rabies vaccine	Aventis Pasteur
	Chiron Behring GmbH & Co.
Rubella virus vaccine, live, attenuated	Merck & Co., Inc.
Smallpox vaccine[b]	Wyeth Vaccines
Tetanus and diphtheria toxoid, adsorbed	Aventis Pasteur, Inc.
	Massachusetts Public Health Biologic Laboratories
Tetanus immune globulin	Bayer Corporation
	Massachusetts Public Health Biologic Laboratories
Tetanus toxoid	Aventis Pasteur, Inc.
Tetanus toxoid, adsorbed	Aventis Pasteur, Inc.
	Massachusetts Public Health Biologic Laboratories
Typhoid vaccine, Vi, polysaccharide	Aventis Pasteur, SA
Typhoid vaccine, live, oral Ty21a	Berna Biotech
Varicella vaccine, live, attenuated	Merck & Co., Inc.
Yellow fever vaccine, live, attenuated	Aventis Pasteur, Inc.

[a] Only protects against types A, B, and E.
[b] Limited availability.

SOURCES: Adapted from FDA (2001b, 2002a), USAMRMC (1999), and Zoon and Goldman (2002).

TABLE 3-3 Selected Vaccines Previously Licensed by FDA but Not Available

Product	Manufacturer
Adenovirus type 4 vaccine, live, oral	Previously manufactured by Wyeth Vaccines (contract awarded to Barr Laboratories by DoD on September 25, 2001)
Adenovirus type 7 vaccine, live, oral	Previously manufactured by Wyeth Vaccines (contract awarded to Barr Laboratories by DoD on September 25, 2001)
Cholera vaccine	Previously manufactured by Wyeth Vaccines
Lyme disease vaccine, recombinant OspA protein	GlaxoSmithKline Biologicals
Plague vaccine	Previously manufactured by Greer Laboratories (still holds license)
Smallpox vaccine	Previously manufactured by Wyeth Vaccines; limited stockpile

SOURCES: Adapted from FDA (2001b, 2002a), USAMRMC (1999), and Zoon and Goldman (2002).

TABLE 3-4 Vaccines Available to U.S. Military Personnel as IND Products

Product	Manufacturer
Botulinum toxoid vaccine, pentavalent	BioPort Corporation
Tick-borne encephalitis vaccine, inactivated	Baxter-Immuno Vertriebs GmbH*

* Although the DoD did administer the tick-borne encephalitis vaccine, inactivated, as an IND product (AFEB, 1993), it does not now have an active IND application for the vaccine and cannot administer it to U.S. military personnel. The vaccine is available in Europe; DoD and the manufacturer are having ongoing discussions about pursuing U.S. licensure for the vaccine (Personal communication, R. Tucker, October 25, 2001; USAMMDA, 2001a).

SOURCES: Adapted from FDA (2001b, 2002a) and USAMRMC (1999).

vaccine, or the inability of manufacturers to meet other regulatory requirements. The last three factors also illustrate the importance of the transition from the production of pilot lots of a vaccine to scale-up of production to a level for clinical use of the vaccine by larger numbers of people. This transition requires that a manufacturer (1) have the technical ability to produce the vaccine, the physical infrastructure to produce the vaccine, and the personnel to divert toward production of the vaccine; (2) possess experience with the regulatory and clinical research affairs needed to successfully license a vaccine; and (3) have the financial motive to engage in the long, arduous, and expensive licensing process in the face

TABLE 3-5 Vaccines Administered as INDs That Are No Longer Being Produced and That Are of Limited Availability

Product	Manufacturer
Argentine hemorrhagic fever (Junin virus) vaccine, live, attenuated	The Salk Institute
Chikungunya virus vaccine, live, attenuated	The Salk Institute
Eastern equine encephalitis vaccine, inactivated	The Salk Institute
Q fever vaccine, inactivated	The Salk Institute
Rift Valley fever vaccine, inactivated and live, attenuated	The Salk Institute
Tularemia vaccine, live, attenuated	The Salk Institute
Venezuelan equine encephalitis vaccine, live, attenuated and inactivated	The Salk Institute
Western equine encephalitis vaccine, inactivated	The Salk Institute

NOTE: All the vaccines listed in this table were initially developed in U.S. Army laboratories. The vaccines underwent further development and scale-up production (at pilot level for investigational use) at the Swiftwater, Pennsylvania, plant of the Government Services Division of the Salk Institute (French and Plotkin, 1999). The plant is now owned and run by Aventis Pasteur, Inc., and does not include a government services division.

SOURCE: Pittman (2000).

of uncertain profits in the end. Time and again, these factors have limited the engagement of the most experienced vaccine manufacturers in the production and licensure of new vaccines, particularly special-use vaccines for use by the military.

CURRENT STATUS OF SELECT MILITARY VACCINE-RELATED RESEARCH PROGRAMS

Table 3-6 provides an overview of USAMRMC's infectious disease research program, showing the Joint Technology Coordinating Group-2 (JTCG-2)[2] priority ranking and the funding available to each research activity. Brief descriptions of the current status of the select vaccine research programs supported by the Military Infectious Diseases Research Program (MIDRP)[3] appear in the following paragraphs.

Malaria Vaccine

Growing resistance to antimalarial drugs has increased the urgency of the malaria vaccine effort. A candidate *Plasmodium falciparum* vaccine—

[2]A discussion of the role and function of the JTCG-2 group is provided in Chapter 2.
[3]A discussion of the role and function of MIDRP is provided in Chapter 2.

TABLE 3-6 USAMRMC Fiscal Year (FY) 2001 Program Priorities, in Decreasing JTCG-2–Assigned Rank, and FY 2000 Investment in Exploratory Research

MIDRP FY 2001 Program Priorities, by JTCG-2–Assigned Rank	FY 2000 Investment in Exploratory Research (millions of $)	JTCG-2 FY 2001 Priority
Malaria vaccines	**5.8**	1
Malaria drug discovery program	4.8	2
Diarrheal vaccines	**4.4**	3
Flavivirus vaccines (includes vaccines against tick-borne encephalitis and dengue viruses)	**2.9**	4
Common diagnostic systems	0.5	5
Malaria genome project	1.4	6
Identification and control of insect vectors	1.6	7
Hepatitis E virus vaccine	**0.9**	8
Polyvalent meningococcal vaccine	**0.5**	9
Vaccine tech	**1.1**	
Hemorrhagic fever and tick-borne encephalitis virus	0.8	10
Hantavirus vaccine	**0.7**	10
Rickettsial diseases	0.7	11
Leishmania research	1.5	Not ranked[a]
Human immunodeficiency virus research	**15.0**	Not ranked[b]
Walter Reed Army Institute for Research overhead	11.0	
Total	53.6	
Total for Vaccines	**31.3**	

NOTE: Program priorities in boldface type represent vaccine-related research.

[a] Gulf War funding.
[b] U.S. Military HIV Research program is one of the Congressional Special Interest Medical Programs assigned to the DoD. Funding for these programs is added to the DoD budget by Congress and is not in the President's budget.

SOURCES: Michael (2000) and Hoke (2000a).

RTS,S[4]—has been in development for more than a decade by SmithKline Beecham Biologicals (now part of GlaxoSmithKline [GSK]) and DoD. RTS,S

[4]RTS,S—"RTS,S is a fusion protein of the carboxyl-terminal half of the *P. falciparum* circumsporozoite protein, which includes part of the central repeating sequence 'R' and major T cell epitopes 'T', and which is fused with the entire surface antigen 'S' of the hepatitis B virus" (Bojang et al., 2001, p. 1927).

combines the hepatitis B virus surface antigen with a circumsporozoite recombinant protein as a virus-like particle formulated with the proprietary adjuvant system AS02. In clinical trials, this vaccine was demonstrated to protect U.S. volunteers against *P. falciparum* malaria and protected 70 percent of semi-immune adults in a field trial conducted in The Gambia, albeit for only 2 months (Bojang et al., 2001; Stoute et al., 1997). The joint efforts of DoD and GSK are enhanced by a partnership with the Malaria Vaccine Initiative at the Program for Appropriate Technology in Health[5] that is enabling evaluation of the vaccine for use in children. A Phase I[6] trial is being conducted in The Gambia, and a Phase II trial is planned for Mozambique in 2002 (GSK, 2001; MVI, 2001). In 1998, a parallel navy program reported the safety of a candidate DNA-based vaccine and its capacity to elicit killer T cells with specificity for malaria peptides. The navy and its partners with which it has Cooperative Research and Development Agreements (CRADAs), Vical and Aventis, are now constructing and testing more complex vaccines. In November 2001, Vical and the U.S. Naval Medical Research Center announced the results of Phase II clinical trials. The trials indicated that the candidate vaccine was safe and well tolerated.

Vaccines Against Diarrheal Diseases

Current research activities directed at protecting military personnel and travelers against the most common types of diarrheal diseases by use of vaccines target some of the bacterial agents of those diseases, in particular, *Campylobacter*, enterotoxigenic *Escherichia coli* (ETEC), and *Shigella*. Several candidate vac-

---

[5]The Malaria Vaccine Initiative was created through initial funding from the Bill and Melinda Gates Foundation.

[6]Prelicensure vaccine trials are divided into three phases. Phase I clinical trials mark the first tests conducted with humans and test the candidate vaccine's safety and immunogenicity in a small number (~20 to 80) of healthy volunteers. Phase II clinical trials also test the vaccine's immunogenicity and safety, but at this phase dose-ranging tests (how much of the vaccine/drug is needed to produce the desired effect) are often initiated. About 100 to 300 subjects are often included in these tests. Phase III clinical trials measure the vaccine's safety, efficacy, and immunogenicity. This phase should generally include thousands of patients and should provide sufficient benefit to risk data to ensure licensure and "provide an adequate basis for product labeling" (FDA, 2001c). Although FDA provides guidelines to steer manufacturers toward licensure of a product (Current good manufacturing practice in manufacturing, processing, packing, or holding drugs; general. 21 C.F.R. § 210 [2001]; Current good manufacturing practice for finished pharmaceuticals. 21 C.F.R. § 211 [2001]; Investigational new drug application [IND]. 21 CFR § 312.20–312.21, subpart B [2001]; Biological products: General. 21 C.F.R. § 600 [2001]; FDA, 1998), the number of individuals included in prelicensure trials of vaccines varies broadly. However, the committee understands that recent FDA requests for prelicensure trials of vaccines to be used in civilian populations have often included 10,000 subjects and in one recent case 60,000 subjects. Efficacy and safety data require use of statistical evaluation to assist in determining the sizes of both types of studies. Safety studies may need to have larger sample sizes than efficacy studies.

cines are in development, although these efforts face many challenges, including the large number of serologically distinct types of these organisms causing diarrhea and the difficulty of inducing a mucosal immune response capable of blocking infection with enteric pathogens. A candidate *Shigella flexneri* vaccine developed at the Institut Pasteur and manufactured at Walter Reed Army Institute of Research (WRAIR) pilot lot production facility was first tested in healthy volunteers at the U.S. Army Medical Research Institute for Infectious Diseases (USAMRIID) in 1996. A larger trial with 100 or more U.S. volunteers is planned for later in 2002. A Phase II clinical trial involving 200 to 300 Bangladeshi children to test the vaccine's efficacy in an environment where the disease is endemic is also planned (USAMMDA, 2001b). Vaccines against other species of the genus *Shigella*—*Shigella sonnei* and *Shigella dysenteriae*—are also being evaluated.

A vaccine designed to protect against ETEC is under evaluation in Egypt, and new vaccines based on microencapsulated ETEC antigens are under development. A *Campylobacter* vaccine is in advanced development, but it is likely that new approaches will be required to make the vaccine more effective. Industry partnerships supporting the research include a DoD Dual-Use Science & Technology program contract with Acambis, Inc. to develop *Campylobacter* and ETEC vaccines (Acambis, Inc., 2001), a CRADA with Antex Biologics, Inc. to develop *Campylobacter* vaccines (USAMMDA, 2001c), and a Small Business Innovation Research program grant from the National Institute of Allergy and Infectious Diseases to develop oral microbead vaccines against diarrhea. Antex Biologics, Inc. is also researching the possibility of a multivalent vaccine to prevent diarrhea caused by *S. flexneri*, *S. sonnei*, *Campylobacter jejuni*, and ETEC (Antex Biologics, Inc., 2001).

Dengue Vaccine

DoD scientists have a long history of experience with dengue vaccines and the development of diagnostic tests for dengue (Innis et al., 1988; Kanesa-thasan et al., 2001; Vaughn et al., 1996). WRAIR and GSK have worked to develop a tetravalent vaccine that is being evaluated in a Phase II clinical trial in Thailand (Innis, 2001; WHO, 2002).

Hepatitis E Vaccine

Epidemiological studies by CDC, the army, the navy, and scientists in Russia, Pakistan, Nepal, and other countries have shown that the hepatitis E virus (HEV) is the most common cause of hepatitis in adults in many developing countries (Clayson et al., 1998). Genelabs, Inc., in collaboration with CDC, isolated and cloned HEV (Genelabs Technologies, 2001). Investigators at the National Institutes of Health (NIH) developed a baculovirus-expressed recombinant protein candidate HEV vaccine in the late 1990s; that vaccine, developed at NIH, is licensed to GSK. Two Phase I clinical trials—one in the United States and one in Nepal—have been conducted through a joint effort of NIH, DoD, Genelabs Technologies, and GSK. A Phase II clinical trial of the vaccine with 2,000 adult volunteers is under way in Nepal (Genelabs Technologies, 2001).

Meningococcal Group B Vaccine

The efforts of investigators at WRAIR led to the development of a quadrivalent polysaccharide meningococcal vaccine that has been recommended for use by selected civilian populations, such as college students (AAP, 2000; CDC, 2000b). Efforts to develop a meningococcal group B vaccine continue, but such a vaccine has proved more difficult to develop (Brundage and Zollinger, 1987; Jódar et al., 2002). Although several promising candidate vaccines based on outer membrane protein processes of the group B meningococcus have proceeded to large-scale field trials, no licensed product is yet available in the United States.

HIV Vaccine

The goal of the U.S. Military HIV Research Program[7] is to develop a vaccine that provides protection against all known subtypes of HIV type 1 (HIV-1) circulating throughout the world. Efforts to date have focused on (1) surveillance for determination of the HIV subtypes infecting U.S. forces; (2) characterization of prevalent subtypes of HIV-1 around the world, including genetic recombinants; (3) collaborative efforts with industrial partners to design vaccine constructs based on a broad array of subtypes, including both those prevalent in the United States and those prevalent in other regions of the world; (4) preparation of field sites in Thailand and Uganda for testing of a vaccine; and (5) conduct of early clinical safety and immunogenicity studies in Thailand, Uganda, and the United States. The program has candidate vaccines—including those that use naked DNA, vectored DNA, and recombinant proteins from HIV subtypes E, A, D, and C—in various stages of development and testing. A Phase III clinical trial, in collaboration with the Ministry of Public Health of Thailand, is scheduled to begin in fall 2002 for evaluation of a vaccine consisting of a canarypox virus vector. The clinical trial will be conducted in Thailand and is expected to last 5 years. In October 2002, DoD will transfer management of the HIV vaccine trial

---

[7]HIV vaccine research is managed as a Congressional Special Interest extramural research program (USAMRMC, 2002a). The research program is a collaborative effort of the air force, army, and navy. The program is headed by WRAIR and research is conducted in collaboration with the Henry M. Jackson Foundation for the Advancement of Military Medicine (U.S. Military HIV Research Program, 2002).

and research effort to NIH to comply with direction from the Office of Management and Budget (NIAID, 2002a).

REGULATORY STATUS OF SPECIAL-USE VACCINES

As mentioned above, DoD maintains a Special Immunizations Program (SIP) within USAMRIID whose mission is to "offer FDA licensed vaccines and investigational new drug (IND) vaccines under informed consent to laboratory workers at USAMRIID, and to other, military, government, or contractor personnel who may be at occupational risk of exposure to highly hazardous pathogenic microorganisms or toxins" (Boudreau and Kortepeter, 2002). SIP administers five FDA-licensed vaccines and nine vaccines with IND status; these are listed in Tables 3-7 and 3-8, respectively. Table 3-9 lists the two vaccines for which CDC is the IND sponsor but which SIP administers to the military.

A number of vaccines that DoD has developed over the years, including the vaccines listed in Table 3-8, have remained at the pilot level of production, with no commercial manufacturers identified. Incentives to pursue full-scale production have been limited primarily because of the geographically limited nature of the diseases that the vaccines were designed to prevent and the limited commercial potential of these products. DoD faces obstacles in keeping these products available to military personnel when the vaccines are needed. Some of the obstacles encountered include the challenges of meeting FDA regulatory requirements, difficulties associated with administering products with IND status, and the increased cost of vaccine development. Significantly, as described in the note to Table 3-8, live, attenuated vaccines against chikungunya virus, Junin virus, and Rift Valley fever virus that were previously available as INDs through SIP no longer have active IND status and thus are not available even for very specialized uses within DoD.

TABLE 3-7 FDA-Licensed Vaccines Used by SIP as of March 2002*

Product	Manufacturer
Anthrax vaccine, adsorbed	BioPort Corporation
Hepatitis B vaccine	GlaxoSmithKline Biologicals Merck & Co., Inc.
Japanese encephalitis vaccine	Research Foundation for Microbial Diseases of Osaka University (Biken)
Rabies vaccine	Aventis Pasteur
Yellow fever vaccine	Aventis Pasteur

* A licensed plague vaccine was previously administered, but it is no longer manufactured.

SOURCES: Boudreau and Kortepeter (2002) and FDA (2001b, 2002a).

TABLE 3-8 Vaccines with IND Status Used by SIP as of March 2002

Product	Year IND Application Filed	Year Last Produced
Eastern equine encephalitis vaccine, inactivated	1967	1992
Q fever vaccine, inactivated	1972	1970
Rift Valley fever vaccine, inactivated	1969	1991
Tularemia vaccine, live, attenuated, LVS strain*	1965	1985
Venezuelan equine encephalitis vaccine, inactivated	1975	1981
Venezuelan equine encephalitis vaccine, live, attenuated	1965	1972
Western equine encephalitis vaccine, inactivated	1984	1972

NOTE: Chikungunya virus vaccine, live, attenuated; Junin virus vaccine, live, attenuated; and Rift Valley fever vaccine, live, attenuated had been included in SIP but are not being administered at present. SIP administered as an IND a tick-borne encephalitis vaccine to U.S. military personnel deployed to Bosnia in 1996. The tick-borne encephalitis vaccine, however, no longer has FDA IND status (Personal communication, R. Tucker, Baxter International, October 25, 2001).

* Clinical use of the vaccine is on hold.

SOURCES: Boudreau and Kortepeter (2002) and Pittman (2000).

TABLE 3-9 Vaccines with CDC-Sponsored IND Status Administered by SIP

Product	Year IND Application Filed	Year Last Produced
Botulinum pentavalent toxoid	1979	1995
Smallpox vaccine (Dryvax®)	2001	1982

NOTE: The army also has a separate IND application (Army BB-IND #3723) on file for botulinum pentavalent toxoid.

SOURCES: Boudreau and Kortepeter (2002) and USAMRMC (1999).

FDA regulations require that a biological product be evaluated for its immunogenicity, safety, and efficacy before licensure. Under current rules, FDA cannot grant a license to a vaccine that has not been shown to be efficacious and safe in clinical trials with humans or for which there is no robust laboratory evidence that indicates that the vaccine offers the same protective immunity demonstrated in earlier studies with another vaccine (FDA, 1998). Most of the vaccines that SIP manages are designed to prevent rare infections, natural occurrences of which are unpredictable in everyday settings. To a large extent, that may preclude the possibility of completing conventional clinical efficacy trials with these vaccines.

The ability to conduct experimental challenge tests is severely limited or absolutely prohibited by well-accepted ethical rules guiding human experimentation. Therefore, it would be very difficult to meet the current FDA requirements for licensure for these vaccines.

Two FDA rules address the difficulty of providing sufficient evidence of efficacy for these vaccines. A rule finalized as the committee completes this report allows the use of data from animal studies as surrogates for human-study data when it is not feasible to conduct tests with humans. The rule concerns the constraints on the testing of the efficacy of a vaccine and does not address the requirement to demonstrate the safety of the product in large numbers of humans (FDA, 2002c). A second rule—subpart H: Accelerated approval of new drugs for serious or life-threatening illnesses[8] —permits accelerated approval of new drugs for serious or life-threatening illnesses. It states that "FDA may grant marketing approval for a new drug product on the basis of adequate and well-controlled clinical trials establishing that drug product has an effect on a surrogate endpoint."

To detect relatively low frequency adverse events related to vaccine administration, tests need to be conducted with substantial numbers of subjects, making the demonstration of safety and efficacy not only difficult but also costly. Several published estimates from the pharmaceutical industry and others indicate that approximately 60 to 75 percent of vaccine development costs occur in the late stage of product development (Greco, 2001; Monath, 2000). These and related issues are discussed further along with the recommendations in Chapter 4.

Current regulations preclude the use of products with IND status without adherence to extant regulations applicable to clinical research with experimental products.[9] This includes the submission to FDA of certain information pertaining to the product and the proposed clinical studies, prior approval by an independent institutional review board, the collection of informed consent, and detailed recordkeeping.[10] The myriad procedures and documentation steps can be difficult—if not impossible—to adhere to during military operations.

---

[8]Accelerated approval of new drugs for serious or life-threatening illnesses. 21 CFR § 314.500–314.560, subpart H (2001).

[9]Investigational new drug application (IND). 21 CFR § 312.20–312.21, subpart B (2001); Informed consent of human subjects. 21 CFR § 50, subpart B (2001).

[10]From DoD Directive 6200.2: Use of Investigational New Drugs for Force Health Protection (DoD, 2000).

> 4.8.1. Notice Requirement for IND Use: When using an IND for force health protection, DoD Components shall provide prior notice to personnel receiving the drug or biological product of the following:
>
> 4.8.1.1. That it is an IND (including specific information on whether it is approved by FDA and/or whether it is unapproved for its applied use).
>
> 4.8.1.2. The reasons the IND is being used.

In 1990, at the request of DoD, FDA published an interim rule addressing DoD's concerns about the use of products with IND status in combat situations. The interim rule allowed the FDA commissioner to waive the informed consent requirement when such a waiver was requested by the Assistant Secretary of Defense for Health Affairs. Application of the rule was restricted to the "use of an investigational drug (including an antibiotic or biological product) in a specific protocol under an investigational new drug application" and was "limited to a specific military operation involving combat or the immediate threat of combat."[11] The rule was applied during the Gulf War, allowing the use of pyridostigmine bromide and a botulinum toxoid vaccine to protect against the potential use of weaponized biological or chemical agents (Rettig, 1999).

When service members returned from the Gulf War deployment and reported medically unexplained symptoms, many questioned the safety and efficacy of the vaccine and drug products used during the war and the wisdom of DoD's use of the interim rule. These perceptions, which may have been different had there been credible evidence of the actual use of chemical or biological weapons by forces opposing U.S. and allied personnel, sparked changes in the government's policy regarding the IND waiver. In part because of concerns that grew out of the use of the interim rule during the Gulf War, the U.S. Congress passed an amendment to the Defense Authorization Act for FY 1999[12] that vests solely with the president the authority to waive the informed consent requirement. Accordingly, FDA revoked the 1990 interim rule and established a new interim final rule outlining the limited circumstances in which the president could waive the informed consent requirement: "if the President finds obtaining informed consent (1) not feasible; (2) contrary to the best interests of the members; or (3) not in the best interests of national security" (FDA, 1999, p. 54181).

DoD was again criticized for administering a product with IND status without close adherence to the FDA guidelines when it used the tick-borne encephalitis (TBE) vaccine in the Bosnian conflict. For many years, the military had

---

4.8.1.3. Information regarding the possible side effects of the IND, including any known side effects possible as a result of interaction of the IND with other drugs or treatments being administered to such personnel.

4.8.1.4. Other information as required to be disclosed by the FDA.

4.8.2. Information to Providers for IND Use: DoD Components shall ensure that healthcare providers who administer the IND or who are likely to treat members who receive the IND receive the information identified in sections 4.8.1.3 and 4.8.1.4 above.

4.8.3. Record Keeping on Use of IND and Notice Requirement. DoD Components shall ensure that medical records of personnel who receive an IND accurately document the receipt of the IND and the notice required by section 4.8.1 above.

[11] Informed consent of human subjects. 21 CFR § 50, subpart B (2001).

[12] Strom Thurmond National Defense Authorization Act for Fiscal Year 1999. P.L. 105-261 (1998).

administered the TBE vaccine to U.S. personnel who inspected military sites in the Soviet Union, where TBE is endemic. The vaccine, developed by scientists from Austria and the United Kingdom, had been widely used in Europe but had not been licensed for use in the United States. In 1993, the Armed Forces Epidemiological Board (AFEB) was asked to evaluate and make a recommendation regarding the use of the TBE vaccine (for which the Army held an IND application). AFEB recommended that the vaccine against TBE be used "under IND protocol with informed consent" to protect military personnel with significant potential for exposure to TBE (AFEB, 1993). In 1996, the Assistant Secretary of Defense for Health Affairs outlined, based on input provided by USAMRMC and the surgeons general, DoD policy regarding the use of a vaccine against TBE. The policy instructed that the TBE vaccine should be offered to "personnel at very high risk of tick exposure" and that it should not be used to routinely immunize all DoD personnel (ASD[HA], 1996). DoD offered the TBE vaccine to soldiers deployed to areas in Bosnia known to be affected by tick-borne encephalitis. To receive the vaccine, however, individuals had to volunteer to participate in a study of the IND product and, accordingly, to provide written informed consent.

An investigation by the General Accounting Office into the Army's recordkeeping practices during the Bosnian conflict (GAO, 1997) found that nearly one-fourth of the immunizations against TBE in Bosnia were not properly documented. FDA, also, found "significant deviation" from the guidelines related to the use of a product with IND status in DoD's use of the TBE vaccine in Bosnia (FDA, 1997b). Although DoD officials "acknowledged faulty recordkeeping," they maintained that IND guidelines were followed (Gillert, 1998). The TBE vaccine is no longer available to U.S. military personnel as a product with FDA IND status.

The sequence of events outlined above highlights the difficulties inherent in complying with FDA rules related to an IND product and conducting well-documented clinical trials of investigational vaccines among military personnel engaged in combat or participating in peacekeeping duties under hazardous conditions. They also point out the difficulties that commanders face when they must confront the rules and regulatory practices that are in place when they are deploying forces into situations that are likely to expose those forces to infectious disease threats for which licensed vaccines may not be available.

4

Recommendations with Accompanying Analysis of Limitations Imposed by Current Department of Defense Structure for Managing Acquisition of Vaccines Against Infectious Diseases

Substantial shifts have occurred in the geopolitical, budgetary, and psychological framework within which the Institute of Medicine (IOM) committee that has prepared this report began its work 2 years ago. The September 11, 2001, terrorist attacks heightened the nation's sense of vulnerability, and contamination of the U.S. mail with anthrax spores focused the public's attention on bioterrorism and infectious disease threats. To the Department of Defense (DoD), however, the reality of infectious disease threats predated this recent national interest. DoD's longstanding interest in the use of vaccines to protect military personnel against infectious disease threats is reflected in this committee's charge as well as in DoD's separate request to an expert panel led by Franklin Top, Jr., (DoD, 2001d) for advice on its vaccine production capability. These two reports and the recent statement by the IOM Council (IOM, 2001) encouraging the creation of a National Vaccine Authority share a common sense of urgency in suggesting that changes are needed in the processes by which the government acquires vaccines. At the same time, the President's fiscal year (FY) 2003 budget proposal, the heightened public perception of infectious disease threats, and the attention now focused on biodefense provide unparalleled opportunities for change and set the stage for DoD to act.

Thus far in this report, the committee has presented mostly factual, descriptive information about the need for vaccines, their use in the U.S. military, and the organizational procedures through which DoD advances a vaccine from the point of recognizing the need for a vaccine to making it available for use by military personnel. Here, the committee presents its discussion of those organizational, procedural, and scientific components and provides its analysis of how the pieces might be made to fit better and how the overall process of vaccine acquisition might be improved. Wherever possible, the committee cites specific evidence to support its conclusions. However, in a number of instances no such data were available and the committee was forced to rely on the perceptions of those interviewed by the committee or on indirect evidence, often in combination with the past experiences of committee members in their interactions with both military and civilian vaccine acquisition systems. In such cases, the committee has made every effort to note the lack of hard evidence supporting its contention.

Protecting the health of military personnel is essential to national security. The committee presented in Chapter 1 historic evidence that infectious diseases have posed significant threats to the health of the nation's armed forces. Chapter 3 describes those vaccines that are available to the military for the prevention of infectious diseases. A review of the data presented in this report (e.g., Chapter 3) makes it clear that no vaccine is available for many of the infections that have previously posed problems for U.S. forces on overseas deployments (e.g., dengue, diarrhea, and tick-borne encephalitis, to name a few of those listed in Table 1-2). Thus, it is clear that infectious diseases remain a major concern even as the twwenty-first century unfolds. The considerable number of overseas deployments of U.S. forces on warfighting and peacekeeping missions in recent years suggests that the risk of exposure of military personnel to both naturally acquired and intentionally released infectious agents remains real and present.

Vaccines are often the most cost-effective way to protect individuals from infectious diseases, but their value is easily overlooked both within the civilian public health sector and within the military community. For example, a successful antiballistic missile defense system may provide dramatic evidence for its utility when it destroys an incoming warhead, but a safe and effective vaccine leaves no trace of its success when the immune response that it has engendered in the immunized soldier thwarts the early stages of a potentially lethal infection and prevents an incapacitating illness or death. On the basis of its review of the circumstances surrounding the loss of the adenovirus vaccines and the lack of an available licensed plague vaccine (Table 3-3) and (until very recently) an anthrax vaccine, as outlined below, the committee believes that DoD must assign a higher priority to vaccine acquisition than it has in the past.

For the purposes of this discussion, the committee defines *acquisition* as the process by which DoD ensures that appropriate vaccines are available for the protection of its forces. This process represents a continuum extending from the first recognition of need, to the setting of priorities, to the maintenance of a technology base permitting internally conducted or externally contracted product-oriented research, advanced product development, and clinical studies leading to licensure (whether or not DoD is in partnership with an industrial entity), as well as the establishment and maintenance of effective manufacturing facilities and, ultimately, the procurement (purchase) and stockpiling of vaccine for use by DoD for protection of members of the U.S. armed forces.

The committee's main conclusion is that DoD's current vaccine acquisition procedures, coupled with its complex annual budgeting process, significantly hamper its vaccine acquisition activities and thwart effective coordination with vaccine manufacturers. The evidence that led the committee to this conclusion is laid out in the pages that follow. These limitations result in an inability to develop the vaccines that are needed (as evidenced by the large number of vaccines listed in Table 3-5 that are no longer being actively developed for protection of the armed forces), instability in essential vaccine-related research programs (which is reflected in wide fluctuations in budget authority, as described below), and the failure to have available for immediate use those vaccines that are critical for the protection of military personnel, as cited above. The ultimate cost of this inefficient acquisition process is that military readiness is placed at risk. Some militarily important vaccines are not available, in whole or in part, because of poorly aligned acquisition processes and an inadequate commitment of financial resources rather than because of unmet scientific or technological hurdles. This is particularly true for the vaccines listed in Table 3-5, including, for example, the attenuated Junin virus (Argentine hemorrhagic fever) vaccine, for which evidence supporting substantial clinical efficacy has been amassed in a trial carried out among civilian populations in South America (Maiztegui et al., 1998).

DoD's current approach to vaccines originates with the best intentions, involves skilled individuals, millions (but not sufficient millions) of dollars, and intricate planning. Nevertheless, the committee's assessment after hearing from many of those involved in the acquisition process, as well as several executives from the companies that manufacture vaccines, is that the current vaccine acquisition process has limitations that make the path from basic research to procurement and use of vaccines both inefficient financially and cumbersome. These limitations result in occasional outright failure (as in the case of the loss of the adenovirus vaccines) and unacceptable delays (in the case of the anthrax vaccine) in vaccine acquisition. The lack of vaccines when and where they are needed risks the success of future military operations and the health of personnel and potentially places national security in jeopardy.

The committee's recommendations cover four broad aspects of the acquisition process:

1. Organization, authority, and responsibility
2. Program and budget
3. Manufacturing
4. Regulatory status of special-use vaccines

After first presenting its nine recommendations in Box 4-1, the committee provides a discussion, building its case with examples and presenting the reasoning that has resulted in each recommendation.

BOX 4-1
Committee Recommendations

Organization, Authority, and Responsibility

The committee recommends that the Department of Defense:

1. Combine all DoD vaccine acquisition responsibilities under a single authority within DoD that attends to the entire spectrum of responsibility—from definition of a potential threat against which a vaccine is needed through research and development, advanced product development, clinical trials, licensure, manufacture, procurement, and continued maintenance of manufacturing practice standards and regulatory compliance.

2. Consolidate the infrastructure, funding, and personnel for DoD programs for the acquisition of vaccines against weaponized biological agents and naturally occurring infectious diseases.

3. Ensure that there is an effective, ongoing senior advisory group—one providing perspectives from both within and outside of DoD—to assess program priorities and accomplishments, to act as a proponent for vaccines and other infectious disease countermeasures, and to maintain active relationships with current science and technology leaders in the academic, government, and corporate sectors.

Program and Budget

The committee recommends that the Department of Defense:

4. Provide budget resources commensurate with the task.

5. Actively encourage the development, distribution, and use of a well-defined and validated research priority-setting mechanism. Such a mechanism could involve the use of prioritized, weighted lists of infectious disease threats and formal scenario-planning exercises and would require the use and synthesis of infectious disease surveillance and epidemiologic information.

6. Include programming goals that ensure greater strength and continuity in the science and technology base for the full spectrum of infectious disease threats, including research related to the epidemiology of infectious diseases, the nature of protective immunity, and both early and advanced vaccine product development.

7. Leverage DoD research efforts by building greater interactions and an effective formalized coordinating structure that links DoD research activities to vaccine development activities carried out by the Department of Health and Human Services and other public and private groups.

Manufacturing

The committee recommends that the Department of Defense:

8. Work toward improving manufacturing arrangements to ensure consistent vaccine availability by addressing issues related to long-term commitments, predictable volumes and prices, indemnification, and intellectual property issues. These arrangements should include consideration of the development of vaccine-specific partnerships between the federal government and individual private manufacturers, a consortium of private vaccine manufacturers, and government-owned, contractor-operated vaccine production facilities.

Regulatory Status of Special-Use Vaccines

The committee recommends that the Department of Defense:

9. Vigorously seek a new paradigm for the regulation of special-use vaccines that remain in investigational new drug application status with the Food and Drug Administration and that have no reasonable prospects for licensure under the current rules. The new paradigm should take into account the circumstances of the vaccine's anticipated use in setting requirements for the demonstration of safety and efficacy.

ORGANIZATION, AUTHORITY, AND RESPONSIBILITY

Early in the committee's deliberations, one DoD representative attempted to clarify the DoD process for setting vaccine research and development priorities with an illustrative slide, presented here as Figure 4-1 (and earlier as Figure 2-1). It clearly conveys the complex gauntlet awaiting the potential acquisition of a new vaccine from the time of the first conception of its need through the late stages of development. Figure 4-1 also vividly demonstrates the absence of a single organizational locus of authority and responsibility for that process. Not only is no individual in charge, but too many individuals and entities are responsible for other, unrelated activities in addition to their responsibilities for vaccines and the development of effective countermeasures against infectious disease threats. The committee believes that DoD's vaccine acquisition program does not—and cannot—work effectively with its management structured in this fashion.

Perhaps the best example of how such diffuse management arrangements thwart effective vaccine acquisition is the loss of the adenovirus type 4 and 7 vaccines that the U.S. military used very effectively for many years to prevent acute respiratory disease among trainees. The committee heard from representatives of both DoD and the vaccine manufacturer (Wyeth) concerning the events that led up to the decision by the latter to cease manufacture of the vaccine because of its inability to make changes to its manufacturing facility required by the Food and Drug Administration (FDA) under the terms of its existing contract with DoD. What the committee heard was the inability of the manufacturer to identify any single point of authority within DoD that was sufficiently knowledgeable about the issues and sufficiently empowered to make changes in the contract with the manufacturer necessary to maintain vaccine production. No single entity in DoD had sufficient breadth of authority or responsibility to approve further research and development or to authorize modifications to the manufacturing facility once the vaccine had become licensed, even though this meant that production of the vaccine would cease and that future procurement would not be possible. The end result was the recurrence of serious adenovirus respiratory infections among basic trainees, a problem that continues to the present.

This particular issue was the subject of an interim report (IOM, 2000a; also provided as Appendix A to this report) released by the IOM committee that has prepared this report. Although one cannot be certain that a consolidation of all responsibility for vaccine acquisition within a single authority in DoD would have prevented the loss of these vaccines, the committee is convinced that the disjointed authority for advanced vaccine development and vaccine procurement that exists within DoD contributed significantly to the lack of the additional investment required for continued production of this vaccine.

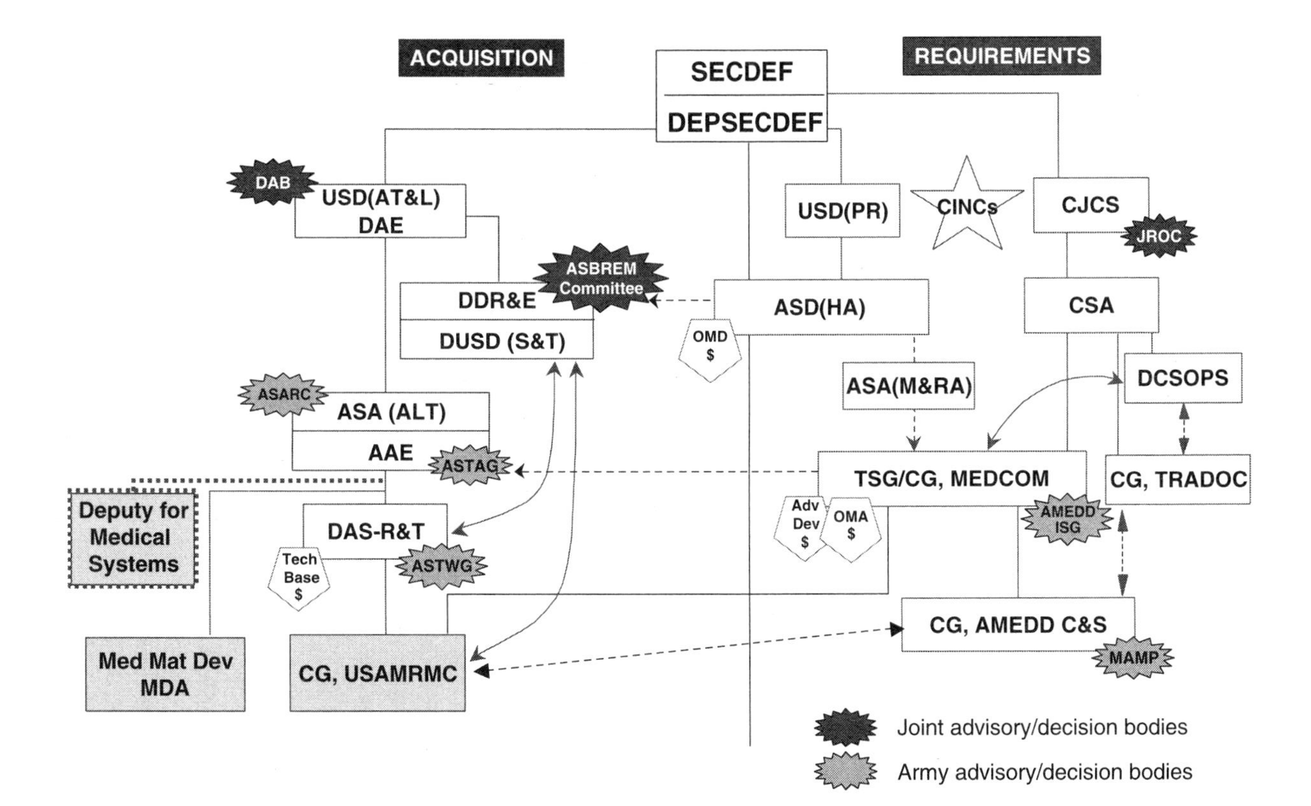

FIGURE 4-1 Military infectious disease-related research, development, and acquisition activities: USAMRMC interfaces with army and Office of the Secretary of Defense organizations. The acronyms and abbreviations included in this figure are identified in the caption to Figure 2-1 of this report. SOURCE: Glenn (2000).

Another expert committee commissioned by DoD recently reached a similar conclusion (DoD, 2001d). Soon after IOM constituted the committee that has authored this report at the request of the U.S. Army Medical Research and Materiel Command (USAMRMC), the Deputy Secretary of Defense directed the Acting Assistant Secretary of Defense for Health Affairs (ASD[HA]) and the Director of Defense Research and Engineering to form a group, chaired by Franklin Top, Jr., and charged it with a task—based on the requirements outlined in P.L. 106-398—that significantly overlapped that of the IOM committee. Working independently and with different emphases, the two committees identified similar systemic problems and arrived at similar recommendations to address them, including the need for centralized and coordinated management and strengthened, supportive expert advice.

These committees are not the first to note organizational and procedural problems within the DoD's acquisition processes. The DoD Reorganization Act of 1986 called on DoD to "reduce and streamline the defense bureaucracy" (Republican Policy Committee, 1986). DoD, itself, has recognized the need to reform its acquisition system—agency wide. In 1994, the Secretary of Defense released a report entitled *Acquisition Reform: Mandate for Change* outlining the need to change the acquisition system. It noted, "The problem is that the DoD acquisition system is a complex web of laws, regulations, and policies. . . While each rule individually has (or had) a purpose for its adoption, and may be important to the process as a whole, it often adds no value to the product itself, and when combined, contributes to an overloaded system that is often paralyzed and ineffectual, and at best cumbersome and complex" (DoD, 1994, pp. 5, 6). In 2001, DoD again addressed the inefficiency of the acquisition system in its *Quadrennial Defense Review Report*, which notes that "two major institutional processes—the planning, programming and budgeting system and the acquisition process—create a significant amount of the self-imposed institutional work in the Department. Simplifying these processes will support a streamlining of the entire organization [the Department of Defense]" (DoD, 2001c, p. 52). The General Accounting Office (GAO), in testimony before Congress on February 27, 2002, notes that despite DoD's heavy dependence on acquisition—"close to $100 billion annually to research, develop, and acquire weapon systems and tens of billions more services and information technology" (GAO, 2002, p. 1)—its acquisition system is inefficiently managed. GAO studies found that responsibility for acquiring services is diffuse and "with little visibility or control at the DoD- or military department level" (GAO, 2002, p. 3). The report notes that DoD "is seeking to adapt the same revolutionary business and management practices that helped the commercial sector gain a competitive edge" (GAO, 2002, p. 3).

The GAO outlines, in its testimony, several suggested changes that may improve the efficiency of the DoD acquisitions system, including restructuring programs so that requirements and needs are better matched, making sure that decision makers are open to funding the lifecycle of a product, and assuring that those making decisions—in terms of time and money spent on a product—are sufficiently knowledgeable about the product and are persons vested with the authority "to make informed tradeoff decisions" (GAO, 2002).

Diffuse Management Responsibility

As detailed above, no identifiable decision maker within DoD has the responsibility and authority for vaccine acquisition. No single organizational agent within DoD drives the vaccine acquisition system or acts as a galvanizing motivator. No single organizational unit within DoD has the authority to address problems arising with licensed products to maintain product availability.

Because no single authority within DoD oversees the vaccine acquisition effort, the DoD decision-making structure for vaccine acquisition is fragmented at each step of the process, including research, development, production, licensure, and the purchase and stockpiling of vaccines. The fragmentation of these processes hinders the creation of priorities and the acquisition of vaccines that the military needs. It leads to misalignment of resources, creates disparities between vaccine research efforts and relevant military medical operations, and leaves large gaps within the research and development process. It prevents any long-term stability across the many years during which a new vaccine is conceptualized, moves through the preclinical and clinical research stages, and finally, is licensed. Furthermore, just as budgetary authority is disjointed, so is program authority. Even the various research and development components—technology base and advanced development—do not share an effective prioritization mechanism. The committee was unable to identify a single list of priorities for vaccine acquisition that each of these separate DoD entities involved in the vaccine acquisition continuum uses. This disconnect can result in the misdirection of resources.

Consolidating responsibility and authority for the acquisition of vaccines within a single organizational entity or vaccine authority would provide a seamless process by which DoD could acquire vaccines to provide the protection that its forces require. Vaccine acquisition would be enhanced by developing and imposing a common means of prioritization at all levels of the vaccine acquisition effort, by eliminating unnecessary bureaucracy and overlapping, redundant programs, by improving communication among those responsible for different aspects of the vaccine acquisition continuum, by eliminating the waste of program resources, and by managing vaccine acquisition as part of a higher-priority DoD acquisition category (e.g., acquisition category I).

Having expended considerable time in attempting to understand the complexities of the current acquisition process, the committee concludes that DoD should create a single vaccine authority by concentrating responsibility and authority for the entire vaccine life cycle—up to, but not including, policy and clinical decisions concerning the use of vaccines. This entity should be the controlling authority for the acquisition of vaccines and related biological countermeasures and not simply a coordinating body. It should report to the highest levels within DoD. To succeed, this vaccine authority must have the following:

- sufficient authority to influence vaccine development, including adequate budgetary authority with assured funding for operations (such as for the procurement of vaccine products after the research period) and control over any government-owned manufacturing facility, such as the government-owned, contractor-operated (GOCO) facility now being considered by DoD;
- adequate staffing to manage and accomplish all phases of the acquisition process, from priority setting to vaccine research and development, product development, manufacture, and stockpiling;
- personnel with the financial, regulatory, and legal expertise required for all aspects of the vaccine acquisition process integrated within a single office;
- clearly defined relationships with the ASD(HA), the DoD and army offices involved with providing funding for science and technology-related activities and program direction, and the commanding general of USAMRMC;
- a placement in the DoD organizational hierarchy that would allow it to control decisions throughout the vaccine acquisition process and to coordinate decisions related to policies for vaccine use; and
- a stable, adequate, and well-defined budget.

The committee does not have a specific recommendation about where within DoD the operational elements of a single vaccine authority should be placed. It did consider, however, the qualifications and characteristics that a single vaccine authority would possess and how it would work. The committee believes that placement of the vaccine authority at a high level in DoD—at the Pentagon, with the individual in charge of the authority reporting to the highest levels of DoD—is necessary to achieve the task. That organizational placement would not preclude USAMRMC's holding the operational lead for vaccine-related activities.

A November 2001 statement from the IOM Council proposed the development of a somewhat similar authority, the National Vaccine Authority, to confront the problems that the public health sector faces in acquiring limited-use vaccines. The problems that the IOM Council sought to address have much in common with those that are part of the scope of this committee's charge. The IOM Council's statement argues that the creation of a single National Vaccine Authority would help to ensure the availability of vaccines that have limited commercial potentials but that are critically needed for the civilian sector.

Although the committee recommends the creation of a single vaccine acquisition authority within DoD, it recognizes that a vaccine is more than a product that can be built simply to predetermined specifications, purchased on bid from the manufacturing sector, and stockpiled for future use. A vaccine is part of a complex and continuously evolving biological system that is intended to protect the warfighter against an infectious disease. As with any complex system, a vaccine requires constant, well-integrated, and coordinated attention to each facet of its development and maintenance, including disease surveillance, prioritization, research and development, and product refinement in a continuously changing regulatory environment. The committee cites DoD's recent loss of the adenovirus type 4 and 7 vaccines as prima facie evidence of the need for DoD to adopt a systems approach to vaccine acquisition that spans all steps in the acquisition process.

Recommendation 1.
Combine all DoD vaccine acquisition responsibilities under a single authority within DoD that attends to the entire spectrum of responsibility—from definition of a potential threat against which a vaccine may be needed through research and development, advanced product development, clinical trials, licensure, manufacture, procurement, and continued maintenance of manufacturing practice standards and regulatory compliance.

Fragmented Acquisition Programs for Vaccines and Related Biological Countermeasures for Weaponized and Naturally Occurring Infectious Disease Threats

The health of warfighters is at risk both from natural infectious disease threats and from weaponized forms of infectious disease agents that might be intentionally deployed against U.S. forces in combat settings or against civilian populations as agents of terror. Whether natural or weaponized, these two forms of infectious disease threats share much in common. A number of specific pathogens such as those causing plague or hemorrhagic fevers are real and present threats in both contexts. Vaccines have been shown to be capable of providing protection against both natural and weaponized infectious disease threats, drawing in each case on what is a common science and technology base.

The maintenance of separate acquisition programs for threats to military operations from naturally occurring infectious diseases and threats from the intentional and hostile use of biological materials inhibit DoD's ability to make rational decisions related to vaccine acquisition. This complex arrangement arose from DoD's response to congressional direction to consolidate activities related to the acquisition of chemical and biological warfare defense measures. Thus, DoD created the Joint Vaccine Acquisition Program (JVAP) to manage the advanced development of vaccines to protect warfighters against weaponized infectious disease agents. Although well intended, the creation of JVAP has led to new problems. Separate management prevents unified thinking on the acquisition of vaccines such as those against the plague bacterium and the Rift Valley fever virus, each of which could be a natural and a weaponized threat to military personnel. Limited expertise and equally limited budgetary resources are divided in the present scheme, in which DoD has split the responsibility and the authority for the procurement of vaccines against naturally occurring and potentially weaponized infectious disease threats and has established no unifying prioritizing mechanism with which it can manage its limited vaccine development resources. JVAP was intended to streamline acquisition procedures and raise visibility of the need for biodefense products, but these potential benefits have not yet been realized in the acquisition of new vaccine products.

The committee could identify no justification for the separation in the acquisition processes for vaccines against naturally occurring and potentially weaponized infectious disease threats. There is substantial overlap in the agents, technical approaches, and hurdles to be overcome in developing vaccines against the infectious agents that comprise both types of threats. The problem here is not simply that JVAP and USAMRMC's infectious disease program are duplicative. That would be true if both sets of programs were functioning adequately. The reality is that the loss of previously available vaccines and the failure to produce new products indicate that neither program is operating effectively—in part because they are separate. The costs and risks are therefore even higher.

In its second recommendation, the committee seeks to fuse the positive characteristics of JVAP—providing a single point of contact and the authority to use a higher DoD acquisition category—and the medical research expertise and experience of the various components of USAMRMC.

Recommendation 2.
Consolidate the infrastructure, funding, and personnel for DoD programs for the acquisition of vaccines against weaponized biological agents and naturally occurring infectious diseases.

Lack of Sufficient Advisory Structure

The committee recognizes the need for and strongly recommends the creation of an ongoing, senior advisory structure to guide high-level decision making related to the acquisition of vaccines and other medical countermeasures against infectious disease threats. The proliferation of prestigious panels now looking at vaccine acquisition and availability is a potent indication of the lack of a center of strong advocacy and advice at present.

Previously, the Armed Forces Epidemiological Board (AFEB), which reports to the surgeons general of the various services, played a major positive role in military vaccine development. DoD now supports AFEB under the authority and budget of ASD(HA) and also calls upon AFEB for advice concerning a broad range of health care and environmental issues. The committee notes that its present scope is much broader than infectious diseases and that AFEB, as it is constituted at present, has neither a sufficient breadth of expertise in infectious diseases nor enough understanding of the vaccine acquisition process (as outlined in the following paragraph) to fill the specialized advisory role that the committee envisions. With the proposed large increase in FY 2003 funding for biodefense, the need to provide effective advice to the government on how to spend the additional funds for military vaccine needs will, if anything, become more acute. The committee considered two routes that might bolster this function.

The first possible approach would be to reconfigure AFEB so that it includes additional individuals with specialized expertise in tropical and geographic medicine and persons with direct experience in vaccine acquisition, including vaccine research, development, manufacture, and procurement. Although this approach might be favored given the long and prestigious history of AFEB, the addition of these responsibilities might diminish the board's effectiveness in meeting or carrying out its non-infectious disease-related responsibilities. Furthermore, the need for expert external advice concerning DoD's vaccine acquisition activities may be too important to relegate to a subcommittee of AFEB.

Second, as indicated above, AFEB operates under the authority of and reports to ASD(HA). To adequately fulfill the advisory role envisioned for the single vaccine authority by the committee, its advisory body must report to the same level of DoD as the vaccine authority itself, that is, at the highest levels of the department. These factors thus argue in favor of the creation of a new advisory structure, one that the committee believes must be able to function effectively independently of DoD's vaccine acquisition authority and with sufficient scope and authority of its own to ensure the protection of the group's ability to provide unbiased advice and the perception that it is providing such advice. AFEB's role within DoD, its multiple other responsibilities, and its organizational position within the department therefore pose significant challenges.

As a third alternative, DoD could seek an independent (non-DoD) expert body to create and maintain a standing advisory committee under contract.

Any of these options—a restructured and reenergized AFEB, a new advisory committee within DoD, or a newly created, ongoing, independent advisory group outside of DoD—would provide DoD with a group of senior advisers who could evaluate the priorities and operations of a consolidated DoD vaccine authority and who would have the potential to become strong proponents for the work that DoD does regarding vaccines against infectious diseases of military importance. A respected and well-connected champion could help articulate the needs so that the upper echelons of DoD could better understand them and, therefore, within their own fiscal and political constraints and opinions, act to support these important efforts.

Recommendation 3.
Ensure that there is an effective, ongoing senior advisory group—one providing perspectives from both within and outside of the DoD—to assess

program priorities and accomplishments, to act as a proponent for vaccines and other infectious disease countermeasures, and to maintain active relationships with current science and technology leaders in the academic, government, and corporate sectors.

FUNDS AND PROGRAM MANAGEMENT

Funding and program management streams are maintained separately in DoD. Although many of the same organizational units are involved in both processes, the processes themselves are largely distinct. Figure 4-1 illustrates the interactions among the different units of DoD involved in the establishment of requirements and the processes for infectious diseases-related research, development, and acquisition. The complexities of the DoD acquisition system for vaccines and related biological countermeasures against infectious diseases give rise to budgeting and programming difficulties.

These budgeting and programming difficulties are not newly recognized. In 1981 DoD created the Armed Services Biomedical Research Evaluation and Management Committee to "facilitate management coordination, improve information exchange, and accomplish medical research, development, testing and evaluation activities" (DoD, 1996, p. 1–6). In 2001, a panel of experts convened by the Deputy Secretary of Defense found that these problems still linger and should be addressed (DoD, 2001d). The IOM committee concurs.

Complicated Funding Process, Inadequate Funds

Budget decisions are made at many levels of DoD and the Department of the Army and are heavily influenced by the competing priorities of line commanders and various staff components of the armed services and DoD. Segmentation of the military research and development budget makes the process even more complex. The research requirements and budget decisions for the development of components of the technology base follow a pathway very different from that for advanced product development. The budgeting process is further complicated by a split between activities related to naturally occurring infectious diseases and those related to potentially weaponized biological agents that results in research redundancies and fragmented funding, as discussed above. Furthermore, once a vaccine product has been developed and licensed, its procurement and stockpiling for future use are supported by yet other sources of funds. For example, if a vaccine procurement problem that required additional research for its solution were identified but research funding was no longer available, efforts to acquire the vaccine or maintain its availability might languish.

Procurement and maintenance funds, which are provided to the Defense Health Program for ongoing support of health care operations within the military, are not available to support changes in vaccine manufacturing processes or facilities that the supplier may request in response to new regulatory requirements imposed by FDA after licensure of a vaccine. At the same time, funds designated for the technology base and advanced product development may not be deemed suitable for making improvements to a licensed product. This schism in the funding stream is matched by a similar schism in the recognition of responsibility for maintaining effective and acceptable manufacturing processes and facilities by various components of DoD after the licensure of a vaccine. In the case of the adenovirus type 4 and 7 vaccines, for example, this disjointed budgetary process for vaccine acquisition appears to have led directly to the loss of these vaccines by the military. The current process fails to recognize that a vaccine represents a complex biological defense system, not a static product.

It is also noteworthy that the current system produces a budget that is inadequate to effectively support the full spectrum of vaccine acquisition activities that are needed. Although the committee was unable to obtain specific information concerning budgets before 1993, in part because of the difficulties of comparing shifting organizational components over time, it has the strong impression that substantial declines have occurred in terms of the real funding available to support vaccine acquisition activities over the last three decades. The declining budget has resulted in a reduction in the breadth of infectious disease-related research in USAMRMC, which affects both basic and applied research, as well as the product development activities supported by USAMRMC contracts. The number of infectious disease agents that are now actively and credibly studied within DoD laboratories has been reduced over time, as USAMRMC has repeatedly restructured its research programs in an effort to retain adequate funding for what it has considered a core set of priorities. Expertise related to rickettsial and parasitic diseases, for example, has been eroded, and the robust basic and applied infectious disease research programs that spearheaded the development of meningococcal, adenovirus, and hepatitis A vaccines in the 1970s and 1980s have not been replaced by similar, cutting-edge, industry-attracting research and development activities in the 1990s and beyond.

A tangible example of the effect of budget reductions is that USAMRMC is no longer capable of effectively meeting FDA's requirements for maintaining the ongoing investigational new drug (IND) status of a number of encephalitis and hemorrhagic fever virus vaccines, such as the attenuated vaccine developed for protection against Junin virus infections. The very real impact of this lapse in IND status is that DoD will not be able to offer protection even to those research laboratory personnel working with these dangerous agents through the Special Immunizations Program (SIP) managed by U.S. Army Medical Research Institute of Infectious Diseases (USAMRIID), let alone offer protection to troops who could be exposed to these threats in the field. Budget limitations and vaccine availability concerns force USAMRIID to maintain a cap on the number of individuals with access to vaccines administered by SIP (Boudreau and Kortepeter,

2002). The current enrollment cap has effectively made these vaccines unavailable to nonmilitary, academic researchers. Table 3-5 lists eight vaccines that were previously developed and championed by DoD but that are no longer being produced and that, as a result, are available in very limited quantities at present. This list highlights just one facet of the long-term consequences of what the committee senses has been a contraction in the breadth of DoD's vaccine development programs.

Table 4-1 shows the somewhat erratic nature of the funding that has supported the DoD infectious disease science and technology base since 1993. From FY 1993 to FY 2000 there were no sustained increases and the budget clearly failed to keep pace with inflation. A substantial increase in funding in FY 2001 was matched by a decline in funding in FY 2002, demonstrating a lack of the reliable levels of support required to sustain stable, long-term research and development projects such as those required for vaccine acquisition. The record indicates a stagnant investment in funding for vaccines, one that has actually decreased in terms of inflation-adjusted dollars, despite real increases in development costs and regulatory burdens.

The commanding general of USAMRMC spoke to the IOM committee in April 2000 about these budgetary reductions and described a $320 million shortfall in unfunded requirements within USAMRMC over the next 5 years. This included $30 million of army "must-be-funded" items.

As a result of budget constraints that DoD has placed on the science and technology base, it has become increasingly difficult to support the broad technical base needed for the diagnosis, treatment, and prevention of infections that are uncommon among U.S. residents but prevalent elsewhere in the world and that therefore present potential threats to military personnel deployed outside the United States. Erosion of the technology base and the professional expertise available for vaccine development within the armed forces have led to a greater dependence by DoD on the commercial sector to accomplish its vaccine-related aims. This is evidenced by the relatively small number of vaccines being developed by DoD (Table 3-6) and the prominent roles that commercial vaccine manufacturers play in the development of many of these vaccines (e.g., the primary role of GlaxoSmithKline in the development of the hepatitis E vaccine).

The record shows that DoD has no long-term, stable budget to attain and sustain what it needs in terms of vaccine development and production capacity. In addition, discussions between the committee and military decision makers and leaders in the vaccine manufacturing industry make it clear that the uncertain nature of the appropriation process of the federal government makes it difficult to maintain continuous scientific and financial commitment from either within or outside of DoD. As a result, vaccines whose development is technically possible and within the country's grasp scientifically, such as the adenovirus vaccines, or vaccines for which administrative hurdles overshadowed technological obstacles, such as the anthrax vaccine (Zoon, 2000) and a vaccine against plague (FDA,

TABLE 4-1 History of Funding for Science and Technology Base Through the USAMRMC Research Area Directorate for Infectious Diseases, FYs 1994 to 2002 (thousands of dollars)

	2002	2001	2000	1999	1998	1997	1996	1995	1994
Total for infectious diseases	52,507	55,823	41,054	39,282	51,525	45,182	42,717	42,040	41,715
Total for human immunodeficiency virus	16,421	26,838	29,638	19,684	38,367	20,485	24,992	32,028	36,778
Vaccines									
Diarrheal	6,315	8,017	1,382	1,262	1,342	1,608	1,536	1,354	1,547
Malaria	7,318	8,688	5,774	4,856	4,938	5,360	5,343	5,201	4,875
Meningitis	644	903	554	544	493	470	375	451	400
Hepatitis	0	723	906	569	474	910	904	975	1,122
Dengue	3,754	3,791	2,886	2,316	2,349	2,404	3,204	2,350	2,284
Hantavirus	849	1,144	736	761	1,407	1,398	1,480	1,510	1,315
Total for vaccines	**18,880**	**23,266**	**12,238**	**10,308**	**11,003**	**12,150**	**12,842**	**11,841**	**11,543**

SOURCE: Provided by Hoke (2002).

1997c; Greer Laboratories, 2001), have not been available to the military as they are needed.

Budget constraints also limit the ability of USAMRMC to successfully move potential vaccine candidates forward into Phase I and II clinical trials. Budget problems often become more severe at the end of development, when industrial development costs for vaccines generally escalate because of the scale-up of the manufacturing process and the need for clinical trials. Yet, the USAMRMC budget has a severely limited advanced development component. As noted in Chapter 2, advanced development funding for vaccines (excluding the human immunodeficiency virus [HIV] vaccine program) was approximately $5.9 million total in FY 2002 (Hoke, 2002), representing only a very small fraction of the resources that the U.S. military needs to acquire licensed vaccines against a large number of potential infectious disease threats. As a point of reference, the committee notes that the current budget provided for development and acquisition of new smallpox and anthrax vaccines within the Department of Health and Human Services (DHHS), generated in response to the nation's call for greater civilian biodefense activities, totals several $100 million.

As indicated above, in arriving at a budget for the procurement of established vaccines, DoD does not include funds for the resources needed to improve or maintain a vaccine—or, for that matter, the funds needed to revamp a vaccine production system to meet current manufacturing practice standards, which change over time. DoD provides no funds to support changes to the production system needed to respond to new regulatory specifications from FDA. The expense of modernizing the production facilities has not previously been accounted for in the procurement process. The loss of the manufacturing facilities for the adenovirus type 4 and 7 vaccines serves as a specific example of this problem and has led to significant outbreaks of adenovirus disease at training installations and one or more deaths among military recruits.

Obtaining resources sufficient for the purchase of a vaccine—even one that has been developed through the DoD—requires independent funds and decision making from parts of DoD (e.g., through the Defense Health Program) that are not tightly linked to DoD's upstream research and development activities. This provides further evidence of the fragmentation of priority setting and management of the vaccine acquisition process discussed above. To develop a budget, DoD must consider the costs of the entire acquisition process, including costs for the sustained manufacture of a vaccine. To do that, the decision maker must understand the process, where the money is going, and what the expenditure is achieving.

At present, the budget available for the acquisition of vaccines is insufficient for the task. Although the committee recognizes the extreme competition for resources that exists among the many important programs within DoD, it believes that DoD, like the civilian sector, has not invested sufficiently in the acquisition of new vaccines. Explanations may rest, in part, on the great successes achieved in controlling such militarily important diseases as tetanus, meningococcal meningitis, and hepatitis A and hepatitis B and in the almost minimal numbers of casualties from infectious diseases in recent conflicts. This may have led to a sense of complacency concerning the risks posed by naturally occurring infectious diseases. Any complacency about infectious disease threats disappeared, however, in the wake of the anthrax attacks against civilian targets in the fall of 2001.

As the committee drafted this report, the President highlighted the need for a large increase in funding for biodefense-related research and product acquisition in his proposed FY 2003 budget. The committee notes that the growth in funding for the research activities of the National Institutes of Health (NIH) anticipated by the President's proposed budget will likely lead to the discovery of novel immunization strategies and better ways to positively manipulate the human immune system. These advances—coupled with enhancements in relevant areas of the nation's research infrastructure—are likely to provide significant spin-offs for DoD as it attempts to address militarily important naturally occurring infectious diseases.

However, in this atmosphere of increased resources fueled by a heightened awareness of the public's vulnerability to bioterrorist actions, the committee cautions that the United States must sustain its investment in vaccine development activities over many years if it is to successfully develop useful vaccines. There are concerns that the infusion of new funds may be short-lived and thus may fail to meet long-term needs for investment in the critical infrastructure required for vaccine acquisition. The current budget is not adequate to support DoD's acquisition of even a few of the many vaccines needed to protect U.S. forces.

Recommendation 4.
Provide budget resources commensurate with the task.

Fragmented Prioritization and Program Management System

The fragmentation apparent in the budgeting process is also evident in DoD's management system for determining infectious disease-related research priorities. The programming process, for example, suffers because it falters at an important first step: the setting of priorities. The specific infectious disease threats to the armed forces include a broad spectrum of microbial and parasitic organisms. As the global demography and the global ecology change and new infectious diseases emerge, the civilian population of the United States and the U.S. military will continue to need a broad-based research program that is capable of coping with these changes. Setting priorities is an important part of the process of creating program goals.

Resources are not sufficient to develop effective vaccines or biological and medical countermeasures to protect warfighters against all potential infectious disease threats. Given this reality, the need for an effective prioritization mechanism is paramount. At present, USAMRMC does not use a defined process to prioritize the research goals on which it is expending its limited resources. The fact that resources are inadequate to meet all requirements only strengthens the need for a well-defined and validated process that ensures appropriate input from intelligence sources and formal periodic review of priorities in light of the changing international and political landscapes and scientific advances and failures.

The manner in which USAMRMC ranks disease threats, research goals, and specific research projects remains unclear to the IOM committee, despite the many hours that it spent in deliberation and hearing briefings from more than a dozen people. As evidence for the failure of the present system, one could cite the absence of a list comparable to the Category A list[1] of the Centers for Disease Control and Prevention (CDC) to guide the activities of USAMRMC. The task of generating a priority list of infectious disease threats to warfighters rests with the Army Medical Department Center and School. However, the committee found that no such list is available to the Medical Infectious Diseases Research Program. The committee acknowledges that it cannot be certain that having a weighted, prioritized list of disease threats would alter research budget allocation decisions in the short term or the health of troops in the long term. Nevertheless, the committee strongly recommends the development and use of a well-defined and validated priority-setting mechanism. Such a mechanism could be developed by using as tools, for example, weighted, prioritized lists to reduce the chance for misunderstanding.

The U.S. government has sought external guidance in prioritization methodology in the past. The Institute of Medicine itself has issued numerous reports. In the mid-1980s, at the request of the National Institute of Allergy and Infectious Diseases of the National Institutes of Health, the IOM released a two-volume report—covering domestic and international needs—that presented a quantitative methodology for choosing which vaccines to place on accelerated development paths (IOM, 1985, 1986). Estimates of expected health benefits (based on morbidity and mortality) and expected costs (including costs averted by vaccination and the costs of a vaccination program) were compared for a set of candidate vaccines. The authoring committee noted the method's value as a decision tool

[1]In June 1999, CDC convened a group of health experts to assess the threat of potential biological terrorism agents. Using the risk-matrix analysis process, the experts ranked the biological threats according to their potential impact on public health. The Category A list includes agents that would have the "greatest potential for public health impact with mass casualties and [would] require broad-based public health preparedness efforts" (Rotz et al., 2002, p. 226). Some of the biological agents included in the Category A list are those that cause anthrax (*Bacillus anthracis*), plague (*Yersinia pestis*), and smallpox (*Variola major*) (CDC, 2000a; Rotz et al., 2002).

rather than a decision maker. The report illustrated how altering the assumptions and viewpoints quantified in the model would alter the priority rankings.

More than a decade later—and around the time IOM formed the committee issuing this report—the IOM report *Vaccines for the 21st Century: A Tool for Decisionmaking* described a different model for guiding vaccine research direction (IOM, 2000b). The model assigned candidate vaccines to one of four levels based on cost (of research and development, vaccine use, health care, vaccine efficacy and utilization, among others) and quality-adjusted life years (based on, for example, severity of illness and time spent with illness). The report, consistent with its predecessors, emphasized that the cost-effectiveness model "can provide an estimate of the cost of achieving the anticipated health benefit for each of the vaccines studied, but it cannot determine whether that health benefit is worth the cost" (IOM, 2000b, p. 57). The value of the cost-effectiveness model relates to its ability to summarize and compare different kinds of costs and benefits; to clarify assumptions; and to test, using multiple sensitivity analyses, the effect of those and alternative assumptions on the result. Although the report used quality-adjusted life years as its measure of benefit, the analytic technique could be adapted for DoD by examining outcomes such as days unavailable for military duty or other measures of unit combat effectiveness.

A CDC expert panel, in February 2002, published a matrix of "reviewable, reproducible means for standardized evaluations" of civilian effects from potential biological threat agents. The report included a Category A list of select agents that were generated by this methodology (Rotz et al., 2002). The model assigned points based on specific characteristics of a potential agent, such as whether hospitalization would be required for an infected person; what mortality rates would be expected for untreated persons with the infection; whether there would be potential for person-to-person transmission and continued dissemination of the infection (based on various assumptions regarding the route of infection); and the degree of potential public fear or panic as predicted by measures of media-registered public awareness.

A somewhat different approach to priority setting is offered by scenario-planning exercises. Scenario planning promotes the construction of different sets of priorities depending on various possible scenarios that are envisioned for the future. It includes the use of milestones to indicate potential changes in or revalidation of present priorities as advancing time and changing circumstances dictate the greater or lesser likelihood of one future scenario over another. A formal process for scenario planning would be useful in prioritizing threats based on estimated risk exposures and anticipated outcomes in the event of infection and would provide an effective interface between intelligence agencies and the DoD decision makers who manage the vaccine acquisition process. Scenarios are cited by private industry advisors as more than predictive and decision-making tools, providing participants "within the organization . . . a common vocabulary and an effective basis for communicating complex—sometimes paradoxical—conditions and options" (GBN, 2002). Formal scenario-planning exercises compel a group of individuals "to question their broadest assumptions about the way the world works so they can foresee decisions that might be missed or denied" (GBN, 2002). Such planning can provide "a specific point at which the required value judgments are described and incorporated . . . [as] one means of isolating these differences of opinion (which are often incorporated into decision making in an ill-defined way) and determining if they affect the ultimate priorities" (IOM, 1986, p. 2). The end result of scenario planning would be a prioritized list or database of disease threats weighted by potential importance to military operations and subject to periodic review and modification as the geopolitical landscape evolves over time.

An additional level of prioritization might involve determination of scientific opportunities and constraints. DoD should take the weighted, prioritized lists generated by scenario-planning exercises and match these with the scientific opportunities for vaccine development, as well as the anticipated costs and resources required to get a particular product on the shelf. DoD is one of many players in vaccine research and development. Given the magnitude of related research activities in the civilian sector, DoD should use the prioritization process to help refine its research agenda so that it uses its finite intellectual and other resources to its best advantage. For example, DoD might decide that investment in development of a particular vaccine, although strongly indicated by scenario planning because of an anticipated need to protect troops in deployments, would be redundant given ongoing investments in the same research area by industry, NIH, or private foundations. Although the parallel pursuit of different strategies for developing an effective vaccine against a single pathogen by different federal agencies could be justifiable, DoD should examine its entire portfolio of requirements against the spectrum of research conducted outside of DoD when determining where to invest its precious research and development dollars. The committee is not persuaded that DoD has engaged sufficiently in such considerations, which would optimize the management of research and development resources in ways expected to maximize the returns (over both the short term and the long term) on investments.

Whether DoD generates a weighted, prioritized list of disease threats, a weighted list of research priorities, or a formal scenario-planning exercise, the process used in its planning efforts should involve experts from academia, DoD laboratory commanders, DoD preventive medicine officers, and the intelligence community. Furthermore, a prioritization scheme should consider not only vaccines but also other medical countermeasures, including prophylactic drugs. Whatever procedures are followed, the committee recommends that DoD consolidate its prioritization efforts within the framework of the total acquisition process defined above. The product of the prioritizing exercise should be reviewed by the reorganized AFEB or whatever ongoing group of senior advisers is convened in response to Recommendation 3, given above. In addition, the priority-setting process should be iterative and should be performed at least annually within the context of a single DoD vaccine authority. Each year, the output of this prioritization effort would inform decisions on the allocation of the budget among the proposed vaccine research and acquisition items.

Recommendation 5.
Actively encourage the development, distribution, and use of a well-defined and validated research priority-setting mechanism. Such a mechanism could involve the use of prioritized, weighted lists of infectious disease threats and formal scenario-planning exercises and would require the use and synthesis of infectious diseases surveillance and epidemiologic information.

A Declining DoD Technology Base Limits Vaccine Acquisition

Budget competition within DoD pits efforts to build and maintain the military's technology base against projects focused on specific products. Although such a process may produce a list of credible products, it runs the risk of eliminating research in areas low on the list, resulting in a continuing narrowing of the research abilities and scientific horizons of the laboratories. Predicting future infectious disease threats to members of the armed forces is an imperfect science, with emerging disease threats and unpredictable global politics adding to the uncertainty. DoD must have ready access to the pool of knowledge and skills needed to maintain the basic scientific research that is essential for the U.S. military to launch nimble and effective responses to shifting infectious disease threats. The committee thus believes strongly that the maintenance of a broad technology base and an infrastructure for research related to the epidemiology of infectious diseases (e.g., DoD overseas medical research laboratories) is an absolutely necessary adjunct to research and development directed at specific vaccine products.

Although the breadth of the technology base is tied to the magnitude of funding made available for infectious disease-related science and technology, as discussed in Chapter 2, the committee emphasizes that it is also dependent on program priorities. Past successes with effective hepatitis A, Japanese encephalitis, and adenovirus vaccines were built on what appears to have been a more substantial infectious disease technology base within the military than exists now. With the stronger base, DoD did not have to envision these specific successful end products at the inception of the related research programs.

The impact of the elimination of the military draft on the infectious disease technology base over the past several decades may be easy to overlook. Although the committee was unable to obtain specific data supporting the contention that the elimination of the military draft has had an impact on the infectious disease technology base, it holds a strong impression that the shift to all-volunteer military forces in the early 1970s led to a significant reduction in the numbers of young investigators with medical and doctoral degrees entering into and passing through DoD's infectious diseases research laboratories. Historically, those individuals who remained in service formed the core of DoD's professional technology base. In recent years, as many of these individuals have qualified for retirement and have left the service, the scientific cadre within DoD does not appear to have been replenished in a manner that would preserve earlier capabilities. DoD could consider the implementation of loan forgiveness programs to attract highly trained researchers. An example of such a program is NIH's Loan Repayment Program for Clinical Researchers, which repays the education loans of individuals who agree to engage in clinical research at NIH for a minimum of 2 years (AAMC, 2002). A potential unplumbed pool of future infectious diseases vaccine researchers is graduates of the Uniformed Services University of the Health Sciences (USUHS). DoD might consider adding research incentives to its established recruitment programs for clinicians, in addition to creating an M.D./Ph.D. dual degree curriculum at USUHS to create a cadre of military physician scientists with interests in infectious disease control.

An effective system must be dynamic and able to respond to new threats, to maximize the potential of biotechnology, and to use individuals with a diversity of skills and from a diversity of disciplines at all steps in the vaccine acquisition process. Vaccines are complex biological systems. Therefore, an effective process for the acquisition of vaccines must be multidisciplinary in nature, resting on a broadly constituted, diverse technology base extending from disease surveillance and risk assessment technologies to the intricacies of molecular and structural biology, vaccine design and manufacture, and, ultimately, the clinical trials and regulatory science that underlie the licensure and deployment of the final product.

Recommendation 6.
Include programming goals that ensure greater strength and continuity in the science and technology base for the full spectrum of infectious disease threats, including research related to the epidemiology of infectious diseases, the nature of protective immunity, and both early and advanced vaccine product development.

Lack of Integration with Other Public-Sector and with Private-Sector Vaccine Development Efforts

As it is structured at present, the DoD vaccine acquisition program is not well integrated with vaccine-related programs maintained by other public-sector agencies. In fact, the U.S. government has charged no less than five federal agencies in three separate departments with various aspects of the response to infectious diseases. In addition to DoD, DHHS (through CDC, FDA, and NIH), the Department of Veterans Affairs, and, to a lesser extent, other federal agencies carry out activities related to prevention, treatment, and research regarding the control of infectious diseases. Other than broad areas of responsibility, there is no clear articulation of the roles played by each agency in the development of specific vaccines. In addition, with a few exceptions, there is no effective mechanism for the systematic coordination of all such activities across agencies. These exceptions include the Federal Malaria Vaccine Coordinating Committee and the ad hoc creation of formal contracts such as those that exist between DoD investigators and investigators at FDA's Center for Biologics Evaluation and Research on the development of flavivirus vaccines.[2] To the present IOM committee, the lack of an effective mechanism for the systematic coordination of activities results in an uncoordinated response in the development of specific vaccines.

Although the National Vaccine Program Office and the National Vaccine Advisory Committee have statutory responsibilities for the coordination of vaccine acquisition-related activities among federal agencies and despite the extensive work of their members in smoothing the flow of information, they have not assumed the authoritative stature necessary to act effectively. The IOM committee believes that the ineffectiveness is guaranteed by the absence of budgetary authority. This observation strongly informs the committee's own recommendations that the proposed single vaccine authority in DoD have controlling authority for vaccine acquisition, including budgetary authority and adequate funding resources. Such authority is needed to carry a vaccine through the process from an idea to a product that is licensed and continually available.

The parallel efforts under way to create a larger smallpox vaccine stockpile provide a perfect example of how coordination could be improved. A Phase I clinical trial of a cell culture-derived vaccine, developed through the DoD's JVAP, began in April 2002 (Gay, 2002). Meanwhile, DHHS, through CDC, has a contract with a different manufacturer to make a cell culture vaccine to supplement the current stockpile of the previously manufactured smallpox vaccine. The two projects use similar development techniques and are creating essentially the same vaccine. Although DoD is "in continued discussion with the Department of Health and Human Services about collapsing the two individual programs into one nationwide program" (Johnson-Winegar, 2001), the two programs remain distinct. Having multiple manufacturers does provide security for the civilian market (such as for the diphtheria–tetanus product). For special-use vaccines, however, when there are needed vaccines not being developed because of lack of funding, the nation cannot afford that kind of redundancy.

Similar circumstances will occur again and again as it becomes increasingly evident that DoD interests overlap and intersect with civilian interests in estab-

[2]The Laboratory of Vector-Borne Viral Diseases, Division of Viral Products, Office of Vaccine Research and Review at FDA's Center for Biologics Evaluation and Research receives funds from WRAIR for support of research on recombinant flavivirus vaccines (FDA, 2002b).

lishing effective biodefense measures. For example, the infectious disease agents on the CDC Category A list of select agents (CDC, 2000a; Rotz et al., 2002), which NIH is using to guide it in setting research priorities (NIAID, 2002b) as it prepares to receive the $1.8 billion that the President's proposed budget directs for defenses against bioterrorism, overlap extensively with the agents covered by DoD's research programs on biodefense and naturally occurring infectious diseases. In addition, as noted in the Preface to this report the nation's perception of the risks that infectious agents pose as instruments of terror is evolving rapidly, and the committee has written its recommendations against the backdrop of these evolving changes. These exigencies have also figured prominently in the recent decision by the IOM Council to publish a statement regarding the creation of a National Vaccine Authority, as discussed above.

DoD stands to benefit greatly from the infusion of funds to support civilian biodefense activities. DHHS has recognized the need for DoD to play an important role in creating for civilian populations effective vaccine defenses against agents on the Category A list. Because of the more diverse nature of the civilian population in terms of age and underlying health status (NIAID, 2002b), it will be significantly more complex and difficult to meet safety and efficacy requirements for vaccines to protect the civilian population than for vaccines that protect warfighters.

Having presented its reasons for giving a single authority within DoD responsibility for efforts related to the acquisition of vaccines against potential weaponized and naturally occurring infectious disease agents, the committee is aware that separation of the DoD and NIH vaccine acquisition and development programs may also appear arbitrary. A major issue to be addressed as NIH invests its financial resources is the limited numbers of informed infectious disease investigators and vaccinologists who are available to respond to the call for the development of new vaccines. To spread this finite human capital over two or three entities of the federal government could diminish the possibility of success of each. Thus, if the creation of a National Vaccine Authority, as urged by the IOM Council, becomes a reality, the committee encourages those involved to devise a means whereby DoD may contribute to and benefit from that authority's responsibility, management, and budget, while preserving a level of operational independence deemed critical by the committee for DoD to meet its unique requirements.

The committee noted above that there is strong overlap in the infectious disease agents of interest to DoD, either as natural threats or in weaponized formulations, and those of national security concern as potential weapons of terror. Agents on both lists include those responsible for smallpox, anthrax, plague, tularemia, and the viral hemorrhagic fevers. In addition, the science and technologies underlying the development and production of vaccines to protect civilian populations are identical to those underlying the development and production of vaccines to protect military forces. Also, as mentioned above, on a national scale, only limited numbers of infectious disease researchers, virologists, and microbiologists have the experience and technical competence required to work with these agents and others on the Category A list of select agents.

There is a clear need for the close coordination of the vaccine development and production efforts of the civilian sector and those of DoD. All of these efforts are ultimately supported by the same budget and have similar and overlapping, although distinct, goals. DoD interaction with public–private partnerships, such as the International AIDS Vaccine Initiative and the Malaria Vaccine Initiative of the Program for Appropriate Technology in Health, could be better coordinated to everyone's benefit. The challenge will be to develop a mechanism by which DoD maintains an effective voice for its unique needs within the structure of a unified national effort.

Recommendation 7.
Leverage DoD research efforts by building greater interactions and an effective formalized coordinating structure that links DoD research activities to vaccine development activities carried out by DHHS and other public and private groups.

MANUFACTURING

Vaccines succeed only when they are administered to people at risk. No matter how successful the research or skillful the efforts at vaccine development, unless manufacturers produce the vaccines, they cannot prevent disease. Two critical factors in industry's decision to manufacture a vaccine are whether the price that it can charge will outweigh the cost of production and whether the required commitment of corporate resources will mean the loss of significant opportunities for the production of other, potentially more profitable products. Unfortunately, vaccine manufacturing costs are high. DoD has not always succeeded in carefully setting priorities (and, therefore, committing its funds prudently) to ensure that critical vaccines are available when and where they are needed. There are several contributory reasons, as outlined in the following sections.

Government–Industry Relationships and the Economics of Vaccines

One of the reasons underlying past failures in DoD's vaccine acquisition efforts is that DoD lacks an ongoing and coordinated relationship with the small number of remaining large vaccine manufacturers[3] that collectively possess decades of experience in vaccine development, delivery, and other logistics

[3]There are four major vaccine manufacturers: Aventis Pasteur, GlaxoSmithKline, Merck, and Wyeth.

crucial to bringing a vaccine to market quickly and cost efficiently. Meanwhile, the U.S. military has no independent, large-scale manufacturing capability. DoD thus needs what these companies can offer. The fact that some important vaccines that have been developed in the past and for which the science and technology base is well understood—such as the adenovirus and anthrax vaccines—have not been available to the military because the manufacturers ceased production or FDA halted distribution makes clear that this is not a theoretical problem but a real one. DoD needs to create stable incentives and contractual obligations for manufacturers to remain motivated and capable of producing vaccines over the long term. The recent shortages of even those vaccines that are used routinely in the civilian population emphasizes the fragility of the vaccine supply in the United States. Some would consider it a national crisis.[4]

Although the life span of a vaccine may be very long, regulatory science is an evolving field, and changes in manufacturing processes and facilities may be mandated by additional requirements that FDA imposes as it seeks to incorporate new discoveries into its regulatory efforts or to take steps to enhance the safety and efficacy of the products that it regulates. Thus, the costs of product development do not necessarily end with the licensure of a vaccine but potentially continue as long at the vaccine is in use or stored for potential use.

DoD could forge more successful relationships with manufacturers if it better understood the need for long-term commitments as well as the basis on which the vaccine industry works. The vaccine industry is highly regulated by FDA and is dominated by a few large corporations. Those corporations use limited resources to take very large risks when they set out to develop and market a new vaccine. Industry and consulting reports estimate the cost of developing a new vaccine, including facility construction, at $300 to $500 million (DoD, 2001d; IOM, 1993). The costs could be somewhat less if use of a special-use vaccine is to be restricted to military populations, if a single facility could be used to manufacture multiple products, and if smaller Phase II and Phase III safety and efficacy trials were deemed reasonable by FDA given the anticipated scope of use of the vaccine. However, because none of these points can be ensured, the costs of developing a special-use vaccine are still very high. Such expenditures make sense to vaccine manufacturers only when the prospects that they will receive a return on the investment are good—a direct benefit to the shareholder that can justify the investment made by the boards of these publicly held corporations.

One former industry executive estimated that a finished product bringing in less than $100 million a year would not be considered worth the investment required to produce it because its development would tie up the limited technical resources and the expertise of the personnel available to the company for vaccine

[4]CDC's National Immunization Program maintains a list of current vaccine shortages. As of April 22, 2002, six of the nine vaccines recommended for routine childhood immunizations were in short supply (CDC, 2002).

or drug discovery. Such opportunity costs are not acceptable to a vaccine manufacturer who is operating in a competitive external market. Even though the investment may ultimately be profitable, a decision within the company to commit the resources to develop such a vaccine will compete with other opportunities to invest those resources, including opportunities offering potentially much greater returns to shareholders. The industry also shies away from short-term, small projects because they are unstable and disrupt larger operations.

Vaccine development is as complicated for special-use vaccines as it is for those with wider commercial potentials, and thus, with the possible exceptions described above, special-use vaccines are potentially as expensive. An acceptable level of safety must be demonstrated to FDA's satisfaction before licensure. However, the potential financial benefit to the manufacturer from the development of a special-use vaccine—if calculated based on market forces alone—is much less than the potential financial benefit expected from the development of a vaccine with large market potential. In support of these arguments, committee members recalled the absence of a response from even a single major vaccine manufacturer when DoD recently urged the development of a plague vaccine.

The government may pursue several available routes if it chooses to ensure the availability of the special-use vaccines that DoD needs (1) to strengthen and expand its partnerships with individual manufacturers to produce vaccines, (2) to encourage the development of a consortium of major vaccine manufacturers to address this need, and (3) to build its own manufacturing capacity. These approaches are not mutually exclusive, and each is costly and potentially difficult, particularly for products that may have limited markets, if any, within the U.S. civilian population.

Partnerships

Research partnerships between the U.S. military and industrial organizations have resulted in impressive successes—for example, the hepatitis A and Japanese encephalitis vaccines—and experts see promise in other current vaccine efforts supported by industrial partners. The great expansion of Cooperative Research and Development Agreements (CRADAs) signals that more DoD research laboratories are depending on industry partners for support.

The CRADA process successfully creates partnerships with industry, but only for specific projects and only for those that the industrial partner deems to be in its best interest overall. CRADAs may be attractive to industry when they are tied to the development of a vaccine with large commercial potential, such as the hepatitis A vaccine; but they are much less attractive in situations in which the civilian market is limited or absent, as in the case of the plague vaccine. In addition, CRADAs cannot support long-term commitments and, thus, they provide an approach that yields no more than piecemeal results. That dynamic can—and, indeed, does—greatly influence the structure of the vaccine program. However, CRADAs do not fundamentally alter the concerns raised above about the need for the chief executive officer of a large vaccine manufacturer to invest the company's research and development resources in ways that maximize financial returns to the company and the shareholder. In addition, since DoD does not allocate enough advanced development funding to develop all the products that it needs, there is a substantial risk that acquisition efforts will falter in areas where no CRADAs exist.

DoD faces an industrywide lack of interest in the vaccines that it so urgently needs to protect its forces against many infectious disease threats. The committee asked current and past vaccine industry executives to describe the factors that lead manufacturers to avoid the development of vaccines with a limited target population. The views expressed to the committee are summarized here.

- Lower profits. The costs of a vaccine targeted to a limited population are similar to those of a universally recommended vaccine, but the revenues are lower; thus, the profit margin is much lower.
- Higher risk. Even the low potential profit is at risk because the government does not guarantee purchase of the vaccine supply that it has requested.
- Limited resources. All projects (including projects focused on the discovery of potentially profitable new drugs for civilian markets) are in competition with one another for corporate resources. Even a large company does not have sufficient funds or personnel to pursue all products in which it may be interested, and special-use vaccines fare badly when choices are made among competing projects. The diversion of uniquely qualified people to a short-lived project hurts potentially more profitable projects by depriving the latter projects of their expertise and thus represents an unacceptable opportunity cost to corporate entities.
- Safety. Some biological agents that must be cultivated in the process of producing vaccines for the military require expensive biological containment laboratories and present potential risks for workers, despite the use of such facilities as a precaution.
- Regulatory and statutory requirements. Regulatory requirements have become substantially more complex and demanding in recent years. The recent deaths of two individuals during university-sponsored clinical research activities (which were not related to the evaluation of vaccines) have heightened the public's awareness of the risks of such research and have resulted in a substantially intensified degree of oversight and more complex documentation and paperwork requirements for investigators engaging in research with human subjects. These requirements have contributed to the increase in the cost of producing vaccines by current good manufacturing practices and the escalation of expenses involved in shepherding new vaccines through to licensure. These changes in the regulatory burden include tendencies on the part of FDA to ask for larger population sizes in studies examining the risks of adverse events associated with the use of

vaccines, factors that run the risk of driving up substantially the costs of the Phase II and III clinical studies required for licensure. In addition, research involving agents on the Category A list of select agents now involves increasingly complex regulatory and legal oversight because of the USA Patriot Act of 2001,[5] which imposes significant responsibilities on the employer with respect to those employees that it uses in such research, including the exclusion of persons from certain countries, those who have sustained legal difficulties, or those who have received other than honorable discharges from military service. There is the risk that additional rules now under consideration may substantially enhance the burdens associated with research on these agents and thus drive both industrial and academic research laboratories toward less regulated areas of research and vaccine development.

- Indemnification issues. Even when all available precautions are taken, there is still an intrinsic risk that a company may be subjected to litigation as a result of an unexpected adverse reaction to a vaccine. Except for the vaccines covered by the National Vaccine Injury Compensation Program, no federal compensation is available. Without a large revenue stream as insurance, product liability becomes a potentially unacceptable risk. One former industry executive observed that GlaxoSmithKline may not have stopped production of the Lyme disease vaccine, despite substantial liability issues, if the market had been better (Associated Press, 2002).

Liability is further complicated for work with military populations, sometimes characterized as a captive pool. Even when working under strict rules and complying with all FDA requirements, industry would want the federal government to indemnify or provide product liability insurance. Industry cites the compensation claims that followed the mass use of the swine flu vaccine in 1976 as an indication that indemnification is necessary. Insiders cite as a more recent example the government's refusal to indemnify Wyeth for the risk of claims related to the anthrax vaccine as a critical factor in the company's decision not to produce the vaccine during the Gulf War.

In summary, the normal conduct of business for industry involves tendering and cost bidding. However, the process does not operate in this fashion when industry is called on to work with the U.S. military. The DoD makes no continuing, long-term funding commitment to industry, it pays no attention to investments for infrastructure or the need for an acceptable profit margin to support the infrastructure, and makes no commitment to purchase a stable or predictable volume of vaccine over time. Single-phase contracts are unsatisfactory for the planning of construction or for the allocation of scarce human resources by industry, especially when the next phase might go to another entity.

---

[5]Uniting and Strengthening America by Providing Appropriate Tools Required to Intercept and Obstruct Terrorism (USA Patriot Act) Act of 2001, P.L. 107-56:175b (2001).

Industry representatives also voiced expectations that military managers may attempt to influence management decisions that they believe are more properly made by industry and that the budgets proffered by the military will often be insufficient to meet the task requested of industry. The overall impression held by industry, which the committee cannot refute, is that DoD has never been willing to commit sufficient resources to justify the investment that a company would need to make with its own limited resources to produce the products requested. DoD has not been able to adequately fund the infrastructure needed, maintain facilities, or ensure adequate volumes of future purchases. It fails to appreciate the needs for the large industrial vaccine manufacturer to have a stable market for its products and to collect a sufficient margin on its sales to ensure its future growth and survival within a very competitive international marketplace.

The perspectives described above make clear why established, large manufacturers have little interest in developing vaccines that would be used only by the military to protect its forces against infectious diseases and for which a profitable commercial market would not be found in the civilian sector. Meanwhile, although small newcomers to the vaccine industry may be willing to bid on projects of limited scope, such untested partners cannot reliably provide the vaccines that the military requires. This was demonstrated in the recent failure of a small company to provide the plague vaccine.

The committee believes that DoD could better attract the interest of industry by working to mitigate the concerns of industry outlined above. An initial step would be to create a centralized, empowered authority within DoD that would manage all interactions and negotiations with the industry, from early partnerships in research and development to the final procurement and stockpiling of licensed products. This would require a change in military organization such as the establishment of a single vaccine authority, as discussed above in Recommendation 1. The concentrated responsibility would permit the companies to deal with DoD representatives who are both (1) knowledgeable about vaccines and public health and (2) given the authority to commit the necessary resources.

The single vaccine authority could negotiate with active and potential industry partners for multiyear, multiphase contracts (or another suitable financial-legal arrangement) with clear milestones for both parties. These would allow the construction of additional facilities and the maintenance of a cadre of personnel who would produce the requested vaccines for clinical trials and who, after licensure, would manufacture vaccine lots for continued use. The presence of a single vaccine authority within DoD would allow informed consideration of industry requests such as the consideration of cost-plus terms for the research and development phase; fixed-cost contracts for the later development, manufacture, and distribution phases; or, after successful licensing, sale of facilities to industry. The single vaccine authority could also negotiate the financing and future ownership of fixed assets; pricing policy, including price ceilings; incentives—

including, for example, the available tax advantages (for research and development, production, and distribution); and staffing arrangements.

DoD might consider how to make better use of legislation to stimulate production of special-use vaccines—those for which a profitable market base is limited—that are particularly needed and unavailable for military use. U.S. orphan drug legislation has stimulated a notable increase in the introduction of drugs to treat rare diseases (FDA, 2002d; Lichtenberg, 2001), but vaccines—although within the purview of the Orphan Drug Act—have worldwide sales that are relatively small compared with drug sales (AEI, 1997) and have realized smaller gains following introduction of orphan product legislation. For instance, as of 1997 only 8 of 152 approved orphan products were vaccines (Lang and Wood, 1999). The financial incentives offered by the Act, such as tax credits, are not helpful to a tax-exempt government developer but it is unclear to this committee why this legislation has not generated more interest from manufacturers for vaccines for military use. DoD and FDA might explore alternative applications of or changes to current law to encourage private industry (as partners or contractors) and DoD itself to produce special-use vaccines.

DoD must assure potential manufacturers that the costs and benefits are reasonably predictable and somewhat guaranteed. An element in any such a calculation would be a consideration of the opportunity costs, that is, what it would cost industry to develop a product wanted by the military in terms of a reduction in its ability to pursue other, potentially more profitable products. The need for long-term financial support for the maintenance of the availability of critical vaccines cannot be overemphasized. Funds must be committed to maintain production facilities so that current good manufacturing practice requirements are met as necessary. A predictable market would involve the generation and maintenance of a vaccine stockpile, the purchase of guaranteed volumes in the future, and reasonable assumptions regarding pricing.

The lack of a policy that is acceptable to industry regarding indemnification against nonnegligent, adverse reactions is a major obstacle to DoD's ability to attract industry participation in the vaccine acquisition process. DoD should examine the indemnification approaches that the federal government uses for childhood vaccines and civilian employees of the army to see if they might be adapted to use for vaccines for the protection of forces.

DoD and its potential partners in industry must delineate a set of mutually acceptable ground rules for the division of responsibility for the early steps in research, particularly those that lead to proof of principle, and the appropriate handling of the intellectual property that may emerge from joint research endeavors. The burgeoning success of technology management offices within many universities provides strong evidence that the fruits of research can financially benefit laboratories outside the industrial sector. Such benefits are appropriate and should not slow the pace of industrial partnership; rather, they should serve as an impetus for further collaboration between DoD laboratories and industrial vaccine manufacturers. Companies will be attracted to DoD partnerships if the companies are allowed to retain intellectual property rights for use in civilian markets. DoD needs to ensure that the ownership of its intellectual property is being properly and adequately exploited to leverage its research activities. Greater attention to the potential value of intellectual property may be of benefit to the overall DoD research effort.

A Government-Organized Consortium of Major Vaccine Manufacturers

The committee considered the possibility that government–industry partnerships might be managed through an industry consortium that would be formed to deal with the military's requests for special-use vaccines. Such a consortium could be a single industrial vaccine authority working in partnership with the single DoD authority envisioned as described above to distribute the real and intangible costs of military vaccine development among multiple corporate entities in the industry. Such a consortium could field individual requests from DoD and work to locate an interested and qualified manufacturer that would enter into specific discussions with DoD. The mechanism could effectively distribute among the companies that are members of the consortium the opportunity costs involved in investing in the development of vaccines whose manufacture is requested by the federal government. Participation in the consortium could be recognized as a moral imperative, possibly facilitating the acceptance by shareholders of less than optimal business investments made by company boards in the interest of national and international security.

The consortium idea has its proponents and its detractors. Successful examples of different commercial entities with competing interests that have worked together for the benefit of all participants include SEMATECH's experience with semiconductors (SEMATECH, 2002) and Airbus Industrie's experience with the aviation industry (Airbus, 2002). An advantage particularly apt to vaccine development is the ability of a consortium to maximize the use of limited technical and professional expertise and other vaccine research and development resources. Although one can easily envision the problems that would need to be overcome to get competing industrial entities to work together in such a fashion, it seems plausible that the development of special-use vaccines by those with the greatest expertise would be particularly cost-effective. A wariness of the need to share proprietary information is a concern, however.

The idea of a consortium of major vaccine manufacturers has been proposed previously, but the reception to the proposal has been tepid. Several industry executives expressed the opinion, however, that it may now be a reasonable goal given the events of September 11, 2001, and the subsequent anthrax attacks. Any such consortium arrangement would require coordination with the Department of Justice, however, to ensure that consortium members would not be subject to collusion or antitrust investigations for these activities. Presumably, industry's concerns over potential antitrust action by the government would be minimized if the government itself took an active step to organize and promote the consortium.

Government-Owned Contractor-Operated Vaccine Production Facilities

Even with improved relations and successful partnerships between DoD and industry, it is unlikely that the private sector will produce all of the vaccines that the U.S. military needs. For that reason, DoD has explored the development of its own production facility. The Salk Institute operated its Government Services Division (TSI-GSD) at Swiftwater, Pennsylvania, and produced vaccines for DoD until 1995.[6] DoD has not had a manufacturing resource similar to TSI-GSD since then, however. The committee notes that as part of an accelerated program of medical biodefense measures the Defense Authorization Act for FY 2002[7] authorizes DoD to design, construct, and operate a vaccine production facility and to contract for the private production of vaccines there.

Evidence supporting the need for a dedicated manufacturing resource can be found in Table 3-5. Table 3-5 lists eight vaccines that DoD had developed and that TSI-GSD manufactured under contract with the federal government. None of these vaccines are currently in production and thus their availability is severely restricted. None of these vaccines, which were or still are administered as INDs, have commercial markets that have interested or are likely to interest an industrial manufacturer of vaccines to invest in their further development. In these circumstances, if DoD is to make needed vaccines available to its forces, it must have access to a production facility outside of the commercial market.

All the items listed in Table 3-4 and some of those listed in Table 3-5 are likely candidates for production in a government facility. However, the committee emphasizes that regulatory requirements would prevent a single government-owned facility from producing all the vaccines needed. To produce more than one product, DoD would have to build the vaccine manufacturing plants with a modular design that would allow separate manufacturing suites to be used for different types of vaccines.

Government-funded manufacturing facilities could be operated through various models. First, DoD could operate its own facility. Second, if it developed these facilities as government-owned contractor-operated (GOCO) entities, a capable contractor could provide dedicated staff and the facility could operate with a flexibility not allowed by government personnel and budget rules. Third, such facilities could be operated by an industrial consortium, one that could mobilize expertise as required from the ranks of those working within its separate component corporations.

[6]TSI-GSD ceased all operations in 1998.

[7]National Defense Authorization Act for Fiscal Year 2002, P.L. 107-107 (2001).

It is important to acknowledge that use of a GOCO facility would be expensive for at least three reasons. First, manufacturers would exert strong pressure by competing for employees who are highly experienced in the manufacture of vaccines. This means that salaries would need to be competitive with the best in the industry. Despite this, the employment of a highly skilled and experienced private-sector workforce could make up for the higher nominal cost of salaries in terms of efficiency and flexibility and could provide a greater ultimate return on the government's investment. On the other hand, staffing of the GOCO facility by industry would create more competition for scarce expertise.

Second, the use of a GOCO facility would require the federal government to take on the full capital cost of building a production facility. This would be expensive because the facilities would require the use of high-containment technology not only for production but also for the testing of products. Although this approach could drive up the initial investment costs, it could provide corporate entities with an incentive to develop products that might not have sufficient market potential to be profitable otherwise. However, if the federal government makes a decision to invest capital for the construction of vaccine production facilities, an alternative to the GOCO concept would be to work out arrangements with specific companies, in which the federal government would subsidize construction of vaccine production facilities that the manufacturer could use to produce other vaccines when the facility was not in use for the production of vaccines for the U.S. military. This is the mirror image of the suggestion made by some that a GOCO facility might manufacture vaccines for the civilian sector when it was not in use making vaccines for the military, an idea that is anathema to the industry. Because the former situation would shift operations and management costs to the manufacturer, some within the industry are of the opinion that this would be a more efficient and less costly approach than the GOCO approach.

Third, and finally, as with any vaccine manufacturing arrangement, a GOCO facility would receive the strong FDA oversight that is essential to maintaining the efficacy and safety of vaccines. Such oversight is especially vital during the rush to respond to emergencies. The steps that need to be taken to comply with all regulatory requirements are costly, however. In addition, bacterial and viral vaccines provide unique challenges in terms of production and quality and safety control compared with the challenges for other types of pharmaceuticals.

After weighing the available evidence, the committee agreed that DoD should consider establishing a GOCO vaccine manufacturing facility, although it did not believe that the development of such a facility would in any way mitigate the need for DoD to revamp its system for managing the overall process by which it acquires vaccines, including integrating the upstream research and development activities and the downstream production and procurement activities, as outlined above. DoD's fragmented and complex organization for vaccine acquisition must become more efficient and cost-effective, regardless of who operates the actual manufacturing process.

Recommendation 8.
Work toward improving manufacturing arrangements to better ensure consistent vaccine availability by addressing issues related to long-term commitments, predictable volume and price, indemnification, and intellectual property issues. These arrangements should include consideration of the development of vaccine-specific partnerships between the federal government and individual private manufacturers, a consortium of private vaccine manufacturers, and government-owned, contractor-operated (GOCO) vaccine production facilities.

REGULATORY STATUS OF SPECIAL-USE VACCINES

At present, the USAMRMC Special Immunizations Program (SIP) manages the use of 14 vaccines whose future availability is highly endangered. By and large, these vaccines are required for the protection of laboratory workers and other individuals who are at exceptional risk of exposure to the pathogens against which these vaccines are directed. Nine of these vaccines remain unlicensed and are available only under IND status, despite use over the past 30 years in varying numbers of recipients.

Long-term use of these products under continued IND status is problematic. FDA uses IND status to provide a basis for clinical investigations that ultimately lead to the demonstration of the safety and efficacy of a vaccine for use by humans; IND status is thus a step on the pathway toward licensure. The use of IND status to make a vaccine available for a specifically circumscribed but ongoing use without any formal intent of advancing the product through the regulatory pipeline toward the goal of licensure by FDA ignores the intent of an IND classification. The committee believes such practices should end. If DoD needs these vaccines, it needs to establish active development programs for each one.

The committee realizes, however, that there are several substantial obstacles to moving these products from IND status to full licensure by FDA. Demonstration of efficacy may be difficult for these vaccines, because most of the vaccines that SIP manages are designed to prevent rare infections whose natural occurrences are unpredictable. That greatly limits the possibility of completing conventional clinical efficacy trials with these vaccines. The ability to conduct experimental challenge tests with these vaccines is severely limited or absolutely prohibited by well-accepted ethical rules guiding experimentation involving human subjects.

Although FDA recently finalized a rule that allows greater acceptance of efficacy data stemming from animal challenge experiments in making determinations for licensure (FDA, 2002c), the facilities and resources capable of conducting such animal challenge experiments are severely limited. The U.S. government operates only two functional Biological Safety Level 4 (BSL-4) laboratories. Furthermore, studies with animals to demonstrate the efficacy of these vaccines would require more rhesus monkeys than are now available. Increasing those laboratory capabilities would entail considerable expense, although the committee notes that the President's proposed FY 2003 budget may provide the funds to increase the number of BSL-4 facilities. Importantly, however, the costs of completing more extensive efficacy studies with animals with each of the vaccines whose development has been arrested at the IND level could exceed the financial benefit that would be provided if the vaccines were available as fully licensed products. Although the committee recognizes that direct financial benefit is not the only incentive to move from IND status to fully licensed status, it recognizes that cost-effectiveness analyses will be applied to any future programs that are proposed with this intent.

Demonstrating to FDA's satisfaction that these vaccines are sufficiently safe to warrant licensure also poses special problems. For licensure of a product, FDA requires, rightfully, that safety testing involve sufficient numbers of subjects to detect vaccine-related adverse events that might occur at relatively low frequencies. This typically entails the enrollment of 10,000 or more subjects in Phase III clinical trials. These numbers may be justified for prelicensure studies of vaccines that are to be used universally or in large numbers of recipients, but studies of that size are tremendously difficult to conduct for vaccines whose use by DoD is intended to be restricted to small numbers of individuals (such as potentially exposed military personnel) no matter how critical the need.

The committee is aware that if a special-use vaccine were to be licensed by FDA, it could be used outside of the SIP framework, and could be prescribed by a physician for civilian travelers to areas in which the target disease is endemic or in response to an outbreak or a terrorist action. Committee discussion of how to help DoD acquire and maintain special-use vaccines was, therefore, couched in a speculative framework. One approach considered was to base licensure of these special-use products on safety standards that are established with a level of confidence appropriate for the number of intended recipients. For example, in the case of a vaccine with very limited intended use, it might be reasonable to base licensure on the results of safety trials involving much smaller numbers of subjects. A lack of serious adverse events among 300 subjects receiving the vaccine in a clinical study would predict that the vaccine would not produce a serious side effect more than 1 percent of the time. This level of risk might be acceptable if only small numbers of persons were intended to receive the licensed product, particularly if the risk of exposure was substantial and the consequences of infection in a nonimmunized person were severe. Such information concerning the limitations on safety data could be provided as part of package insert and could be used to guide decisions concerning the risks versus the benefits of immunization with that special-use vaccine under specific circumstances. In contrast, when considering the licensure of a vaccine for use in the civilian sector, FDA has consistently sought evidence demonstrating a significantly lower risk of serious adverse events.

Basing safety evaluations on such statistical considerations would not be intended to short-circuit the requirement that licensed products be demonstrated to be safe as well as effective but would aim to establish parameters for safety that would recognize the expected use of the vaccine and the numbers of military personnel who might use it. Limitations on the database supporting safety would therefore need to be considered as part of the policies guiding the use of these vaccines, and these should be considered along with the magnitude and severity of the risk in the absence of immunization. If such a system were put into operation, postlicensure surveillance for adverse events would assume a new level of importance. Importantly, such surveillance is likely to be more feasible, under the conditions of ongoing military operations, than the usual data collection practices involved in the conduct of Phase III studies of a product with IND status. In effect, when standard, large-scale clinical trials of safety cannot be done, rather than prohibit the use of a vaccine that would protect warfighters against highly dangerous pathogens, a better overall strategy would be to use the vaccine according to a new FDA licensure arrangement and conduct active postlicensure surveillance for adverse events.

Yet additional problems face licensure of these vaccines with IND status because the basic research on some of these products was carried out long ago. Some data regarding the process used to manufacture the remaining stocks are not available for FDA review. For other products, it may be necessary to repeat earlier work with newer and more costly technologies.

Despite these financial implications, there are other costs, such as the substantial political costs and the crisis of trust that DoD incurred when veterans objected to the use of INDs during the Gulf War. The concern—which continues today—may have been fueled in part by people equating "investigational" with "unsafe." To avoid such understandable concerns, DoD could work with FDA to define a new category, one that might be suitably placed between IND status and full licensure or that might be a subset of licensure. The committee does not intend to imply that products being used only as an IND and manufactured years ago are either safe or effective (although they may well be). Neither is it dismissive of the critical need to demonstrate the safety and efficacy of vaccines as an important factor in the future protection of warfighters against infectious disease threats. It also recognizes that some IND products may never be suitable for licensure. What it does seek is a pragmatic solution to an impossible set of circumstances that threaten to limit access to useful preventive measures during military operations that entail demonstrable risks of infectious diseases.

The committee suggests that DoD work with FDA to identify options related to the status of vaccines that have not been licensed. Ideas to be considered for a new FDA-sanctioned status extend from a status that is no more than a change in terminology to a status that reflects a wholesale new approach to licensure that recognizes alternative mechanisms to the assessment of the safety and efficacy of vaccines in humans that could be applied to vaccines that are to have only limited routine use or that would be used only under unusual circumstances when the risks of infection are perceived to be exceptionally high. The Defense Authorization Act of 2002[8] mandates a study to examine how the government might accelerate the approval process for biodefense vaccines. Although the committee would have included vaccines against naturally occurring infectious diseases in that scope explicitly, it believes that methods devised to overcome the obstacles to the acquisition of biodefense vaccines will be applicable to vaccines designed to address both kinds of exposures. Achieving success in whichever direction DoD chooses to go will require that scientists effectively communicate a sense of urgency through the program and budget hierarchies.

Recommendation 9.
Vigorously seek a new paradigm for the regulation of special-use vaccines that remain in IND application status with the FDA and that have no reasonable prospects for licensure under current rules. The new paradigm should take into account the circumstances of the vaccine's anticipated use in setting requirements for the demonstration of safety and efficacy.

CONCLUSION

Military scientists have a notable record of accomplishment when it comes to vaccines, including primary or significant roles in the development of vaccines against meningococcal meningitis, hepatitis A, Japanese encephalitis, and other dangerous infectious diseases. Partly because of the success of the DoD research programs, the public and even DoD nonmedical research personnel know little about them or the threats that their products have ameliorated. For example, the prior availability and the benefits of the adenovirus type 4 and 7 vaccines went unnoticed by most training center commanders until the vaccines were lost from the armamentarium and adenovirus disease reemerged at military training installations. By creating a single vaccine authority and a credible advisory board and responsibility over the entire life cycle of a vaccine, from priority setting to stockpiling of licensed products, DoD would enhance not only the effectiveness but also the visibility of its vaccine program, improving the chance of its being provided with a budget of sufficient magnitude to allow it to accomplish its mission. It is a mission of enormous importance. Immunization is often the most effective means of preventing infectious diseases, either in civilian or military populations, and whether caused by naturally encountered infectious agents or purposeful exposures related to bioterrorism or biological warfare.

---

[8]National Defense Authorization Act for Fiscal Year 2002, P.L. 107-107 (2001).

The committee urges DoD to work more aggressively with decision makers in the U.S. Congress and in the executive branch to recognize that infectious disease agents—whether they occur naturally or are weaponized as agents of biological warfare or terror—threaten military operations and, therefore and implicitly, the welfare of the nation. Decision makers must recognize (1) the past, imminent, and possible future successes of vaccines in minimizing those threats; (2) the strong track records and reputations of military research programs in developing vaccines used by the U.S. military as well as in civilian settings; (3) the contributions that DoD's medical research efforts make to foreign policy and national security; (4) the threats to continued vaccine development and the ultimate use of vaccines posed by organizational and fiscal limits; and, consequently, (5) the need for adequate, stable funding and strong management authority. Such changes would allow DoD to optimally advance and exploit the technology available for vaccine development, and to provide the best possible protection of the nation's armed forces against infectious diseases.

In summary, DoD's vaccine acquisition system, despite its distinguished history, diffuses responsibility and is inadequately funded; therefore, it cannot produce the effort required to respond to the magnitude of its task.

References

AAMC (Association of American Medical Colleges). 2002. *Loan Repayment and Forgiveness Fact Sheet.* [Online]. Available: www.aamc.org/students/financing/repayment/nih.htm [accessed May 7, 2002].

AAP (American Academy of Pediatrics). 2000. Meningococcal disease prevention and control strategies for practice-based physicians (Addendum: recommendations for college students). Committee on Infectious Diseases. *Pediatrics* 106(6):1500–1504.

Acambis, Inc. 2000. *Award of Major Contract for Smallpox Vaccine from US CDC.* [Online]. Available: www.acambis.com/cfm/index.cfm?cvar=3news2&news_id=509196687 [accessed October 15, 2001].

Acambis, Inc. 2001. *Acambis Awarded Two US Grants for Vaccine Programmes.* [Online]. Available: www.acambis.com/cfm/index.cfm?cvar=3news2&news_id=21729593 [accessed October 15, 2001].

AEI (American Enterprise Institute for Public Policy Research). 1997. *AEI Book Summary. The Search for New Vaccines: The Effects of the Vaccines for Children Program.* [Online] Available: http://www.aei.org/bs/bs8117.htm [accessed May 24, 2002].

AFEB (Armed Forces Epidemiological Board). 1991. *Coordination of Infectious Disease Research in the Department of Defense.* Washington, DC: Armed Forces Epidemiological Board. [Online]. Available: http://www.ha.osd.mil/afeb/1991/1991-04.pdf [accessed June 12, 2002].

AFEB. 1993. *Tick-borne Encephalitis Vaccine.* [Online]. Available: http://www.ha.osd.mil/afeb/1993/1993-08.pdf [accessed June 7, 2002].

AFEB. 1999. *Vaccines in the Military: A Department of Defense-Wide Review of Vaccine Policy and Practice.* A report of the Infectious Diseases Control Subcommittee of the Armed Forces Epidemiological Board. Falls Church, VA: Armed Forces Epidemiological Board.

AFEB. 2001. *History of the Armed Forces Epidemiological Board.* [Online]. Available: http://www.ha.osd.mil/afeb [accessed January 16, 2001].

Airbus. 2002. *Overview.* [Online]. Available: http://www.airbus.com/about/overview [accessed May 6, 2002].

Antex Biologics, Inc. 2001. *U.S. Army Awards SBIR Grant to Antex to Develop Oral Microbead Vaccines Against Diarrhea.* [Online]. Available: http://www.antexbiologics/news_pr/pr010116.phtm [accessed March 5, 2002].

Associated Press. 2002, February 27. Lyme disease vaccine is taken off of the market. *The Washington Post*. p. A10.

ASA(ALT) (Assistant Secretary of the Army, Acquisition, Logistics, and Technology). 2001. *Army Science and Technology Master Plan*. [Online]. Available: http://saalt.army.mil/sard-zt/ASTMP01/fm.htm [accessed February 11, 2002].

ASD(HA) (Assistant Secretary of Defense, Health Affairs). 1996. *Policy for Tick-borne Encephalitis (TBE) Preventive Measures for US Forces Deployed to Endemic Areas*. [Online]. Available: http://www.ha.osd.mil/policies/1996/tbeoje31.html [accessed March 4, 2002].

Bayne-Jones S. 1968. *The Evolution of Preventive Medicine in the United States Army, 1607–1939*. Washington, DC: Office of the Surgeon General, Department of the Army.

BioPort Corporation. 2002. *BioPort Corporation Gains FDA Approval*. [Online]. Available: http://www.bioport.com/NewsRoom/NewsReleases/BioPort/2002-Jan31.pdf [accessed June 6, 2002].

Bojang KA, Milligan PJM, Pinder M, Vigneron L, Alloueche A, Kester KE, Ballou WR, Conway DJ, Reece WHH, Gothard P, Yamuah L, Delchambre M, Voss G, Greenwood BM, Hill A, McAdam KPWJ, Tornieporth N, Cohen JD, Doherty T for the RTS,S Malaria Vaccine Trial Team. 2001. Efficacy of RTS,S/AS02 malaria vaccine against *Plasmodium falciparum* infection in semi-immune adult men in The Gambia: a randomised trial. *Lancet* 358:1927–1934.

Booz Allen and Hamilton. 1999. *DoD Cooperative R&D Agreements: Value Added to the Mission*. [Online]. Available: http://www.dtic.mil/techtransit/refroom/crada/crada.pdf [accessed May 26, 2002].

Boudreau E, Kortepeter M. 2002. Memorandum from Ellen Boudreau, M.D., Chief, Special Immunizations Program, USAMRIID, and Mark Kortepeter, M.D., Chief, Medical Division, USAMRIID, in response to questions from the Institute of Medicine Committee on a Strategy for Minimizing the Impact of Naturally Occurring Infectious Diseases of Military Importance: Vaccine Issues in the U.S. Military. March 27. Unpublished data.

Brownlee S. 2001, October 28. Clear and present danger. *The Washington Post*. p. W8.

Brundage JF, Zollinger WD. 1987. Evolution of meningococcal disease epidemiology in the U.S. Army. In: Vedros NA, ed. *Evolution of Meningococcal Disease*. Vol 1. Boca Raton: CRC Press. Pp. 6–25.

CDC (Centers for Disease Control and Prevention). 2000a. Biological and chemical terrorism: strategic plan for preparedness and response. Recommendations of the CDC Strategic Planning Workgroup. *Morbidity and Mortality Weekly Report: Recommendations and Reports* 49(RR-4):1–14.

CDC. 2000b. Meningococcal disease and college students. Recommendations of the Advisory Committee on Immunization Practices (ACIP). *Morbidity and Mortality Weekly Report: Recommendations and Reports* 49(RR-7):13–20.

CDC. 2001. Two fatal cases of adenovirus-related illness in previously healthy young adults-Illinois, 2000. *Morbidity and Mortality Weekly Report* 50(26):553–555.

CDC. 2002. *National Immunization Program: Current Vaccine Shortages*. [Online]. Available: http://www.cdc.gov/nip/news/shortages/default.htm [accessed April 25, 2002].

Clayson ET, Vaughn DW, Innis BL, Shrestha MP, Pandey R, Malla DB. 1998. Association of hepatitis E virus with an outbreak of hepatitis at a military training camp in Nepal. *Journal of Medical Virology* 54(3):178–182.

Clinton WJ. 1999. Executive Order 13139. Improving health protection of military personnel participating in particular military operations. *Federal Register* 64(192):54175–54178.

Curtin PD. 1989. *Death by Migration: Europe's Encounter with the Tropical World in the Nineteenth Century*. Cambridge, U.K.: Cambridge University Press.

DA (Department of the Army). 1999. Research, Development, and Acquisition—Army Acquisition Procedures. DA Pamphlet 70-3. Washington, DC: Department of the Army.

DHHS (U.S. Department of Health & Human Services). 2001. *HHS Awards $428 Million Contract to Produce Smallpox Vaccine: Acambis/Baxter Will Produce 155 Million Doses by the End of 2002*. [Online]. Available: http://www.hhs.gov.news/press/2001pres/2001pres/20011128.html [accessed March 4, 2002].

DMM (Directorate of Medical Material). 2002. *DAPA (Distribution and Pricing Agreements) Terms and Conditions*. [Online]. Available: http://www.dmmonline.com/dmmonline/dapa/dapaterms.asp [accessed April 4, 2002].

DoD (Department of Defense). Office of the Secretary of Defense. 1994. *Acquisition Reform: Mandate for Change*. [Online]. Available: http://web1.deskbook.osd.mil [accessed November 24, 2001]

DoD. 1996. *Annual Report to Congress: Nuclear/Biological/Chemical (NBC) Warfare Defense*. Washington, DC: Department of Defense. Pp. 1–6.

DoD. 2000. *Department of Defense Directive: Use of Investigational New Drugs for Force Health Protection (Number 6200.3)*. Washington, DC: Department of Defense. [Online]. Available: http://www.dtic.mil/whs/directives/corres/dir2.html [accessed March 07, 2002].

DoD. 2001a. *Chemical and Biological Defense Program: Research Efforts*. [Online]. Available: http://medchembio.detrick.army.mil/MedBio/MedBioResearch.html [accessed March 7, 2001].

DoD. 2001b. *Contracts—Army, September 26, 2001*. [Online]. Available: www.defenselink.mil/news/sep2001/c09262001_ct461-01.html [accessed October 15, 2001].

DoD. 2001c. *Quadrennial Defense Review Report*. Washington, DC: Department of Defense. [Online] Available: http://www.defenselink.mil/pubs/qdr2001.pdf [accessed October 2, 2001].

DoD. 2001d. *Report on Biological Warfare Defense Vaccine Research and Development Programs*. Washington, DC: Department of Defense. [Online]. Available: http://www.defenselink.mil/pubs/ReportonBiologicalWarfareDefenseVaccineRDPrgras-July2001.pdf [accessed September 7, 2001].

DoD. 2001e. *Requirements Generation System (CJCSI 3170.01B)*. Washington, DC: Department of Defense. [Online]. Available: http://web2.deskbook.osd.mil/default.asp? [accessed November 15, 2001].

DoD. 2002. *Department of Defense Instruction 5000.2, Including Change 2: Operation of the Acquisition System*. Washington, DC: Department of Defense. [Online]. Available: http://www.dtic.mil/whs/directives/ [accessed February 05, 2002].

DSCP (Defense Supply Center Philadelphia). 2002. *Defense Supply Center Philadelphia*. [Online]. Available: http://dscp305.dscp.dla.mil/dmmonline/pharm/vaccines.asp [accessed January 25, 2002].

DTIC (Defense Technical Information Center). 2002. *DOD Dictionary of Military and Associated Terms*. [Online] Available: http://www.dtic.mil/doctrine/jel/doddict/ [accessed May 22, 2002].

Edmondson WP, Purcell RH, Gundelfinger BF, Love JWP, Ludwig W, Chanock RM. 1966. Immunization by selective infection with type 4 adenovirus grown in human diploid tissue culture. II. Specific protective effect against epidemic disease. *Journal of the American Medical Association* 195(6):453–459.

Ellenbogen C. 1982. Infectious diseases of war. *Military Medicine* 147(3):185–188.

Engelman RC, Joy RJT. 1975. *Two Hundred Years of Military Medicine*. Fort Detrick, MD: U.S. Army Medical Department.

FDA (Food and Drug Administration). 1997a. FDA warns Michigan Biologic Products Institute of intention to revoke licenses. [Online]. Available: www.fda.gov/cber/infosheets/mich-inf.htm. [accessed November 1, 2001].

FDA. 1997b. Letter to Edward E. Martin, Acting Assistant Secretary of Defense for Health Affairs from Michael Friedman July 22, 1997. [Online]. Available: http://www.gulflink.osd.mil/library/senate/appx_ee.pdf [accessed April 10, 2002].

FDA. 1997c. Letter to Greer Laboratories. [Online]. Available: http://www.fda.gov/foi/warning_letters/m447n.pdf [accessed February 22, 2002].

FDA. 1998. *Guidance for Industry: Providing Clinical Evidence of Effectiveness for Human Drugs and Biological Products*. Washington, DC: Food and Drug Administration. [Online]. Available: http://www.fda.gov/cber/gdlns/clineff.pdf [accessed February 22, 2002].

FDA. 1999. Human drugs and biologics; determination that informed consent is NOT feasible or is contrary to the best interests of recipients; revocation of 1990 interim final rule; establishment of new interim final rule. 21 CFR § 50 and 312. *Federal Register* 64(192):54179–54189.

FDA. 2001b. *Licensed Establishments and Products: July 17, 2001*. Center for Biologics Evaluation and Research. [Online]. Available: www.fda.gov/cber/ep/part3.htm [accessed September 26, 2001].

FDA. 2001c. *Vaccine Product Approval Process*. [Online]. Available: www.fda.gov/cber/vaccine/vacappr.htm [accessed October 22, 2001].

FDA. 2002a. *Licensed Establishments and Products: January 10, 2002*. Center for Biologics Evaluation and Research. [Online]. Available: www.fda.gov/cber/ep/part3.htm [accessed February 25, 2002].

FDA. 2002b. *Molecular Approaches to Enhance Safety of RNA Virus Vaccines*. [Online]. Available: http://www.fda.gov/cber/research/0700209.htm [accessed March 15, 2002].

FDA. 2002c. New drug and biological products; evidence needed to demonstrate efficacy of new drugs for use against lethal or permanently disabling toxic substances when efficacy studies in humans ethically cannot be conducted. Final rule. 21 CFR § 314 and 601. *Federal Register* 67(105):37988–37998.

FDA. 2002d. Office of Orphan Product Development. *Brief History of the Office*. [Online]. Available: www.fda.gov/orphan/history.htm [accessed February 13, 2002].

FMVCC (Federal Malaria Vaccine Coordinating Committee). 2001. *U.S. Federal Malaria Vaccine Programs: FMVCC's Role*. [Online]. Available: http://www.fmvcc.gov/role.html [December 7, 2001].

French GR, Plotkin SA. 1999. Miscellaneous limited-use vaccines. In Plotkin SA, Orenstein WA, eds. *Vaccines*. 3rd ed. Philadelphia: W. B. Saunders Company. Pp. 728–742.

GAO (General Accounting Office). 1997. *Defense Healthcare: Medical Surveillance Improved Since Gulf War, but Mixed Results in Bosnia*. Report GAO/NSAID-97-136. Washington, DC: General Accounting Office.

GAO. 2002. Statement of Jack L. Brock, Managing Director, Acquisition, and Sourcing Management and Randolph C. Hite, Director, Information Technology Architecture and Systems. *Defense Acquisitions: DoD Faces Challenges in Implementing Best Practices*. Report GAO-02-469T. February 27, 2002 hearing of the Subcommittee on Readiness and Management Support, Committee on Armed Services, U.S. Senate, Washington, DC.

Gay T. 2002. *UK College of Medicine Selected as Site for Smallpox Vaccine Trial*. [Online]. Available: http://www.uky.edu/PR/News/smallpoxvac.htm [accessed May 2, 2002].

GBN (Global Business Network). 2002. *Scenarios*. [Online]. Available: http://www.gbn.org/public/gbnstory/scenarios [accessed June 3, 2002].

Genelabs Technologies. 2001. *Genelabs Technologies Announces Phase II Trial for Hepatitis E Virus Vaccine*. [Online]. Available: http://www.biospace.com/news_story.cfm?StoryID=6344815&full=1 [accessed March 5, 2002].

Gillert DJ. 1998. *DoD: Encephalitis Vaccine Didn't Threaten Soldier's Safety*. [Online]. Available: http://www.defenselink.mil/news/Feb1998/n02051998_9802054.html [accessed October 30, 2001].

Glenn J. 2000. *Research and Development, U.S. Army Medical Research and Materiel Command*. Presented at the Third Meeting of the Institute of Medicine Committee on a Strategy for Minimizing the Impact of Naturally Occurring Infectious Diseases of Military Importance: Vaccine Issues in the U.S. Military, Washington, DC.

Goldenthal K. 2000. *DoD Limited Use Vaccine Development: Challenges and Approaches*. Presented at the Second Meeting of the Institute of Medicine Committee on a Strategy for Minimizing the Impact of Naturally Occurring Infectious Diseases of Military Importance: Vaccine Issues in the U.S. Military, Washington, DC.

Gordon JE. 1958. General Consideration of Modes of Transmission. Medical Department USA. In: Boyd Coates J Jr, ed. *Preventive Medicine in World War II: Communicable Diseases Transmitted Chiefly Through Respiratory and Alimentary Tracts*. Vol. IV. Washington, DC: Office of the Surgeon General, Department of the Army.

Gordon L. 2001. A vaccine manufactured not to be used: contracting for a smallpox vaccine stockpile. In: Ross V, ed. *Social Venture Capital for Neglected Vaccine: Creating Successful Alliances: Proceedings of the Albert B. Sabin Vaccine Institute Seventh Annual Vaccine Colloquium at Cold Spring Harbor, New York*. New Canaan, CT: The Albert Sabin Institute. Pp. 89–91.

Gray GC, Callahan JD, Hawksworth AW, Fisher CA, Gaydos JC. 1999. Respiratory diseases among U.S. military personnel: countering emerging threats. *Emerging Infectious Diseases* 5(3):379–387.

Gray GC, Goswami PR, Malasig MD, Hawksworth AW, Trump DH, Ryan MA, Schnurr DP for the Adenovirus Surveillance Group. 2000. Adult adenovirus infections: loss of orphaned vaccines precipitates military respiratory disease epidemics. For the Adenovirus Surveillance Group. *Clinical Infectious Diseases* 31(3):663–670.

Greco M. 2001. *Push and Pull Strategies*. First Meeting of the GAVI Partners, November 20–21, Noordwijk. [Online]. Available: http://www.vaccinealliance.org/reference/ppt/greco.ppt [accessed February 20, 2002].

Greer Laboratories. 2001. Letter regarding availability of the plague vaccine. October 11.

GSK (GlaxoSmithKline). 2001. *Pediatric Clinical Trial for GlaxoSmithKline Malaria Vaccine to Begin Next Month in The Gambia*. [Online]. Available: www.worldwidevaccines.com/public/bio/pressr.asp [accessed October 5, 2001].

Hoke CH Jr. 2000a. *Military Infectious Diseases Research Program Background*. Presented at the First Meeting of the Institute of Medicine Committee on a Strategy for Minimizing the Impact of Naturally Occurring Infectious Diseases of Military Importance: Vaccine Issues in the U.S. Military, Washington, DC.

Hoke CH Jr. 2000b. *Requirements revisited*. Presented at the Fourth Meeting of the Committee on a Strategy for Minimizing the Impact of Naturally Occurring Infectious Diseases of Military Importance: Vaccine Issues in the U.S. Military, Washington, DC.

Hoke CH Jr. (Director, Military Infectious Disease Research Program, USAMRMC). 2002. Response to request for information from Institute of Medicine Committee on a Strategy for Minimizing the Impact of Naturally Occurring Infectious Diseases of Military Importance: Vaccine Issues in the U.S. Military. January 9. Unpublished data.

Innis B. 2001. *GSK's Commitment to Vaccine Research: Taking Fear From the Future*. [Online]. Available: http://www.worldwidevaccines.com/public/bio/Dominican/Bruce_Innis.ppt [accessed March 5, 2002].

Innis BL, Eckels KH, Kraiselburd E, Dubois DR, Meadors GF, Gubler DJ, Burke DS, Bancroft WH. 1988. Virulence of a live dengue virus vaccine candidate: a possible new marker of dengue virus attenuation. *The Journal of Infectious Diseases* 158(4):876–880.

IOM (Institute of Medicine). 1985. *New Vaccine Development: Establishing Priorities, Vol. I Diseases of Importance in the United States*. Washington, DC: National Academy Press.

IOM. 1986. *New Vaccine Development: Establishing Priorities, Vol. II Diseases of Importance in Developing Countries*. Washington, DC: National Academy Press.

IOM. 1992. *Emerging Infections: Microbial Threats to Health in the United States: Summary*. Washington, DC: National Academy Press.

IOM. 1993. *The Children's Vaccine Initiative: Achieving the Vision.* Washington, DC: National Academy Press.

IOM. 2000a. *Urgent Attention Needed to Restore Lapsed Adenovirus Vaccine Availability: Letter Report.* Washington, DC: National Academy Press.

IOM. 2000b. *Vaccines for the 21st Century: A Tool for Decisionmaking.* Washington, DC: National Academy Press.

IOM. 2001. *Statement of the Council of the Institute of Medicine.* [Online]. Available: http://www.iom.edu/IOM/IOMHome.nsf/Pages/Vaccine+Development [accessed November 5, 2001].

IOM. 2002. *The Anthrax Vaccine: Is it Safe, Does it Work?* Washington, DC: National Academy Press.

Jódar L, Feavers IM, Salisbury D, Granoff DM. 2002. Development of vaccines against meningococcal disease. *Lancet* 359(9316):1499–1508.

Johannes L, McGinley L. 2001, October 19. Search for better anthrax vaccine increases. *The Wall Street Journal.* p. A9.

Johnson-Winegar A (Deputy Assistant to the Secretary of Defense for Chemical/Biological Defense). 2000. *Department of Defense Anti-Biological Warfare Vaccine Acquisition Program.* Statement at the April 14, 2000 hearing of the Subcommittee on Personnel, Armed Services Committee, U.S. Senate, Washington, DC.

Johnson-Winegar A (Deputy Assistant to the Secretary of Defense for Chemical/Biological Defense). 2001. *Biowarfare Defense Vaccines.* Statement at the October 23, 2001 hearing of the Subcommittee on National Security, Veterans Affairs and International Relations, Committee on Government Reform, U.S. House of Representatives, Washington, DC.

JSLD (Joint Staff, Logistics Directorate–J-4). Director for Logistics and Director for Medical Readiness. 1999. *Force Health Protection.* [Online]. Available: http://www.dtic.mil/jcs/j4/divisions/mrd/fmp.htm [accessed May 23, 2002].

JVAP (Joint Vaccine Acquisition Program). 2001. *Joint Vaccine Acquisition Program.* [Online]. Available: www.jpobd.net/jvap01.htm [accessed February 21, 2001].

Kanesa-thasan N, Sun W, Kim-Ahn G, Van Albert S, Putnak JR, King A, Raengsakulsrach B, Christ-Schmidt H, Gilson K, Zahradnik JM, Vaughn DW, Innis BL, Saluzzo JF, Hoke CH Jr. 2001. Safety and immunogenicity of attenuated dengue virus vaccines (Aventis Pasteur) in human volunteers. *Vaccine* 19(23-24):3179–3188.

Kassalow JS. 2001. *Why Health is Important to U.S. Foreign Policy.* [Online]. Available: http://www.cfr.org/public/pubs/Kassalow_Health_Paper.html [accessed October 8, 2001].

Kelley PW. 1999. Emerging infections as a threat to multinational peacekeeping forces. *Médicine Tropicale (Mars)* 59(2):137–138.

Lang J, Wood S. 1999. Development of orphan vaccines: an industry perspective. *Emerging Infectious Diseases* 5(6):749–756.

Lichtenberg FR. 2001. *The Effect of New Drugs on Mortality from Rare Diseases and HIV.* Working Paper 8677. Cambridge, MA: National Bureau of Economic Research. [Online]. Available: http:www.nber.org/papers/w8677 [accessed May 30, 2002].

Maiztegui JI, McKee KT Jr, Barrera Oro JG, Harrison LH, Gibbs PH, Feuillade MR, Enria DA, Briggiler AM, Levis SC, Ambrosio AM, Halsey NA, Peters CJ. 1998. Protective efficacy of a live attenuated vaccine against Argentine hemorrhagic fever. AHF Study Group. *The Journal of Infectious Diseases* 177(2):277–283.

McNeill KM, Hendrix RM, Lindner JL, Benton FR, Monteith SC, Tuchscherer MA, Gray GC, Gaydos JC. 1999. Large, persistent epidemic of adenovirus type 4-associated acute respiratory disease in U.S. Army trainees. *Emerging Infectious Diseases* 5(6):798–801.

Michael R. 2000. *Prioritization of Research: MIDRP 2001.* Presented at the Second Meeting of the Institute of Medicine Committee on a Strategy for Minimizing the Impact of Naturally Occurring Infectious Diseases of Military Importance: Vaccine Issues in the U.S. Military, Washington, DC.

Monath T. 2000. *Industry Involvement in Federal Vaccine Development and Procurement Efforts.* Presented at the Second Meeting of the Institute of Medicine Committee on a Strategy for Minimizing the Impact of Naturally Occurring Infectious Diseases of Military Importance: Vaccine Issues in the U.S. Military, Washington, DC.

MVI (Malaria Vaccine Initiative). 2001. *Clinical Trials of Advanced Malaria Vaccine Candidate Expand to Mozambique.* [Online]. Available: www.malariavaccine.org [accessed January 10, 2001].

NAMRU-2. Undated. *Early Warning Outbreak Recognition System (EWORS)—Collaboration between the Institute of Health Research and Development, Ministry of Health, Indonesia and U.S. Naval Medical Research Unit 2.* Pamphlet presented to subcommittee of the Institute of Medicine Committee to Review the Department of Defense Global Emerging Infections Surveillance and Response System, Indonesia, October 2000.

NIAID (National Institute of Allergy and Infectious Diseases). 2000. *The Jordan Report 2000.* Washington, DC: National Institutes of Health. [Online]. Available: http://www.niaid.nih.gov/publications/pdf/jordan.pdf [accessed February 7, 2001].

NIAID. 2002a. *NIAID Phase III HIV Vaccine Trial to Determine Correlates of Protection Will Not Proceed. Phase III Trial in Thailand to Determine Efficacy Will Be Supported by NIAID Through a Combined NIAID-DoD Program.* Washington, DC: National Institutes of Health. [Online]. Available: http://www.niaid.nih.gov/newsroom/releases/phase3hiv.htm [accessed March 15, 2002].

NIAID. 2002b. *The Counter-Bioterrorism Research Agenda of the National Institute of Allergy and Infectious Disease (NIAID) for CDC Category A Agents.* Washington, DC: National Institutes of Health.

NIC (National Intelligence Council). 2000. *The Global Infectious Disease Threat and Its Implications for the US* (Report NIE-99-17D). [Online]. Available: http://www.cia.gov/cia/publications/nie/report/nie99-17d.html [accessed June 3, 2002].

NIH (National Institutes of Health). 2002a. *National Institutes of Health: Press Release for the FY 2003 President's Budget.* [Online]. Available: http://www.nih.gov/news/budgetfy2003/2003NIHpresbudget.htm [accessed March 15, 2002].

NIH. 2002b. *National Institutes of Health, Office of AIDS Research.* [Online]. Available: http://www.nih.gov/od/oar/public/pubs/fy2003/fy2003cj.pdf [accessed June 14, 2002].

NSTC (National Science and Technology Council), Executive Office of the President. 1996. Presidential Decision Directive NSTC-7: Emerging Infections. NSTC-7.

NVPO (National Vaccine Program Office). 2001. *Committees and Working Groups of the NVPO.* [Online]. Available: http://www.cdc.gov/nvpo.committee.htm#iag [accessed December 11, 2001].

Ognibene AJ. 1987. Medical and infectious diseases in the theater of operations. *Military Medicine* 152(1):14–18.

Paul JR, Gardner HT. 1960. Viral Hepatitis. Medical Department USA. *Preventive Medicine in World War II: Communicable Diseases Transmitted Through Contact or By Unknown Means.* Vol. V. Washington, DC: Office of the Surgeon General, Department of the Army.

PhRMA (Pharmaceutical Research and Manufacturers of America). 2000. *2000 Survey: New Medicines in Development for Infectious Diseases.* Washington, DC: Pharmaceutical Research and Manufacturers of America.

Pittman P. 2000. *Status of Limited Use Vaccines in the Military.* Presented at the Second Meeting of the Institute of Medicine Committee on a Strategy for Minimizing the Impact of Naturally Occurring Infectious Diseases of Military Importance: Vaccine Issues in the U.S. Military, Washington, DC.

Republican Policy Committee. 1986. *Senate Record Vote Analysis, 99th Congress: DoD Reorganization.* [Online]. Available: www.senate.gov/~rpc/rva/992/99293.htm [accessed May 26, 2002].

Rettig RA. 1999. *Military Use of Drugs Not Yet Approved by the FDA for CW/BW Defense*. RAND Report #MR-1018/9-OSD. Santa Monica, CA: RAND Institute. [Online]. Available: http://www.rand.org/publications/MR/MR1018.9/ [accessed November 17, 2001].

Rotz LD, Khan AS, Lillibridge SR, Ostroff SM, Hughes JM. 2002. Report summary: public health assessment of potential biological terrorism agents. *Emerging Infectious Diseases* 8(2):225–230.

Sanchez JL, Binn LN, Innis BL, Reynolds RD, Lee T, Mitchell-Raymundo F, Craig SC, Marquez JP, Shepherd GA, Polyak CS, Conolly J, Kohlhase KF. 2001. Epidemic of adenovirus-induced respiratory illness among US military recruits: epidemiologic and immunologic risk factors in healthy, young adults. *Journal of Medical Virology* 65(4):710–718.

Secretaries of the Air Force, Army, Navy, and Transportation. 1995. *Air Force Joint Instruction 48-110, Army Regulation 40-562, Bureau of Medicine & Surgery Instruction 6230.15, Coast Guard Commandant Instruction M6230.4E. Immunizations and Chemoprophylaxis*. [Online]. Available: http://www.dtic.mil/whs/directives/ [accessed November 15, 2001].

SEMATECH. 2002. *Corporate Information: History*. [Online]. Available: http://www.sematech.org/public/corporate/index.htm [accessed April 2, 2002].

Scott B. 2000. *Requirements Determination*. Presented at the Third Meeting of the Institute of Medicine Committee on a Strategy for Minimizing the Impact of Naturally Occurring Infectious Diseases of Military Importance: Vaccine Issues in the U.S. Military, Washington, DC.

Stoute JA, Slaoui M, Heppner DG, Momin P, Kester KE, Desmons P, Wellde BT, Garcon N, Krzych U, Marchand M. 1997. A preliminary evaluation of a recombinant circumsporozoite protein vaccine against *Plasmodium falciparum* malaria. RTS,S Malaria Vaccine Evaluation Group. *New England Journal of Medicine* 336(2):86–91.

Top FH Jr., Grossman RA, Bartelloni PJ, Segal HE, Dudding BA, Russell PK, Buescher EL. 1971. Immunization with live types 7 and 4 adenovirus vaccines: safety, infectivity, antigenicity, and potency of adenovirus type 7 vaccine in humans. *The Journal of Infectious Diseases* 124(2):148–154.

TRADOC (U.S. Army Training and Doctrine Command). 1986. *Operational and Organizational (O&O) Plan for Medical Defense Against Infectious Disease*. Fort Monroe, VA: U.S. Army Training and Doctrine Command.

TRADOC. 1999. *Force Development—Requirements Determination*. TRADOC pamphlet 71-9. [Online]. Available: http://www-tradoc.army.mil/tpubs/pams/p71-9/1999/p71-9.html [accessed November 24, 2001].

USAMMDA (U.S. Army Medical Materiel Development Activity). 2001a. *USAMMDA Information Paper—TBE*. [Online]. Available: http://www.armymedicine.army.mil/usammda/info335.pdf [accessed November 24, 2001].

USAMMDA. 2001b. *USAMMDA Information Paper—Shigella*. [Online]. Available: http://www.armymedicine.army.mil/usammda/info363.pdf [accessed November 24, 2001].

USAMMDA. 2001c. *USAMMDA Information Paper—Campylobacter*. [Online]. Available: http://www.armymedicine.army.mil/usammda/info196.pdf [accessed November 24, 2001].

USAMRMC (U.S. Army Medical Research and Materiel Command). 1999. *Medical Products for Supporting Military Readiness: Vaccines & Drugs (GO Book)*. Washington, DC: Department of Defense.

USAMRMC. 2001a. *USAMRMC: Command Brochure*. [Online]. Available: http://mrmc-www.army.mil/ [accessed November 24, 2001].

USAMRMC. 2001b. *USAMRMC: Command Organizations*. [Online]. Available: http://mrmc.detrick.army.mil/ [accessed November 24, 2001].

USAMRMC. 2001c. *USAMRMC: Command Overview*. [Online]. Available: http://mrmc.detrick.army.mil/hdqoverview.asp [accessed November 24, 2001].

USAMRMC. 2001d. *USAMRMC: Organization Chart*. [Online]. Available: http://mrmc.detrick.army.mil/hdqorgchart.asp [accessed November 24, 2001].

USAMRMC. 2002a. *CSI Research: Research Area Directorates*. [Online]. Available: http://mrmc.detrick.army.mil/crprads.asp [accessed February 28, 2002].

USAMRMC. 2002b. *USAMRMC: Organization Chart*. [Online]. Available: http://mrmc.detrick.army.mil/hdqorgchart.asp [accessed June 13, 2002].

U.S. Military HIV Research Program. 2002. *Overview*. [Online]. Available: http://www.hivresearch.org/overview/index.html [accessed May 27, 2002].

Vaccine Stockpile Strategy. 2002. Vaccine Stockpile Strategy Cost Implications Should Be Considered—NVAC. *"The Pink Sheet": Prescription Pharmaceuticals and Biotechnology* 64(14):31.

Vaughn DW, Hoke CH Jr, Yoksan S, LaChance R, Innis BL, Rice RM, Bhamarapravati N. 1996. Testing of a dengue 2 live-attenuated vaccine (strain 16681 PDK 53) in ten American volunteers. *Vaccine* 14(4):329–336.

WHO (World Health Organization). 2002. *Dengue Fever*. [Online]. Available: http://www.who.int/tdr/diseases/dengue/dengue-poster.pdf [accessed March 5, 2002].

Widdus R. 2001. Public-private partnerships for health: their main targets, their diversity, and their future directions. *Bulletin of the World Health Organization* 79(8):713–720.

Zoon KC. 2000. Statement of Kathryn Zoon, Ph.D., Director of the Center for Biologics Evaluation and Research, Food and Drug Administration, on the anthrax vaccine to the Committee on Armed Services, U.S. Senate, Washington, DC.

Zoon KC, Goldman B (Director, Center for Biologics Evaluation and Research, Food and Drug Administration; Special Assistant, Associate Director for Regulatory Policy, Office of Vaccines Regulation and Research, Food and Drug Administration). 2002. Memorandum in response to questions from the Institute of Medicine Committee on a Strategy for Minimizing the Impact of Naturally Occurring Infectious Diseases of Military Importance: Vaccine Issues in the U.S. Military. February 11. Unpublished data.

Appendixes

Appendix A

Urgent Attention Needed to Restore Lapsed Adenovirus Vaccine Availability

A Letter Report

Committee on a Strategy for Minimizing the Impact of
Naturally Occurring Infectious Diseases of Military Importance:
Vaccine Issues in the U.S. Military

Medical Follow-up Agency

INSTITUTE OF MEDICINE
Washington, D.C.

Urgent Attention Needed to Restore Lapsed Adenovirus Vaccine Availability

A Letter Report

November 6, 2000

Major General John Parker
Commanding General
U.S. Army Medical Research and Materiel Command
Fort Detrick, MD 21702-5012

Dear General Parker:

In April 2000, the Institute of Medicine of the National Academies convened an expert committee to advise the U.S. Army Medical Research and Materiel Command on the management of natural infectious disease threats to the military. The Committee on a Strategy for Minimizing the Impact of Naturally Occurring Infectious Diseases of Military Importance: Vaccine Issues in the U.S. Military will issue its complete report in January 2002. At its initial three meetings, the committee reviewed the failure of the Department of Defense (DoD) to maintain a supply of the adenovirus vaccine as an example of the problems DoD faces regarding the licensure, manufacture, and maintenance of special use vaccines. Production of this vaccine ceased in 1996 and stocks were depleted in 1999. What the committee heard was extremely disconcerting with respect to the threat that the lack of this vaccine now poses to the health of recruit populations. The committee submits this interim letter report today with a sense of extreme urgency in an effort to reinforce the view that there is a critical need for the DoD to expeditiously reestablish a process for the licensure, manufacture, purchase, and distribution of the adenovirus vaccine to military personnel undergoing recruit training activities.

The committee found:

- that the adenovirus vaccine is urgently needed to control the epidemic respiratory disease that has caused much morbidity among recruits in the past, and now once again threatens the health and even the lives of military trainees; since acute pulmonary infection due to adenovirus is a nearly unique occupational risk of the military trainee, it is imperative that DoD take rapid and effective action to once more eliminate this preventable disease;
- that the short-term, $14 million Defense Health Program commitment to acquiring an adenovirus vaccine is insufficient to stimulate the interest of capable commercial vaccine manufacturers; and
- that the existing acquisition and procurement systems within DoD are not structured to ensure continuing availability of limited use vaccines.

The committee recommends:

- that a much greater sense of urgency be placed on reacquiring an effective adenovirus vaccine;
- that a significantly larger and long-term commitment be made to restore and maintain the ongoing availability of adenovirus vaccine; and
- that the DoD not only evaluate the cause(s) underlying this serious procurement system failure, but also make a clear commitment to the changes necessary to prevent similar breakdowns in the future. In its final report to you, this committee will address system issues in depth in an attempt to help the Department of Defense define and then resolve the problem.

The basis for these findings and recommendations is presented in the text that follows.

INTRODUCTION

Capping 30 years of military medical research, the licensure of adenovirus type 4 and type 7 oral vaccines was a great success story. Epidemics of severe acute respiratory disease (ARD) had been a leading cause of hospitalization among recruits in Army, Navy, and Marine Corps training installations. In 1971, the first year of widespread use, adenovirus vaccines prevented an estimated 27,000 military hospitalizations. The risk of the severe ARD epidemics of the 1950s and 1960s was abolished. The impact of the vaccines, including a reduced need to recycle trainees who missed critical training due to hospitalization, as well as savings in the costs of medical care, made the vaccines extremely cost effective.[1]

As a result of a series of decisions that were made beginning in 1984 by Food and Drug Administration regulators, the manufacturer, and DoD officials, the sole manufacturer, Wyeth-Lederle Vaccines, ceased production of adenovirus vaccines in 1996.[2] Discussions between DoD and the manufacturer between 1984 and 1996 failed to lead to a mutually acceptable agreement that would have allowed continued vaccine availability. No alternative source of the vaccine has been found. The military was the only purchaser of adenovirus vaccine and limited its use to recruits in training operations; no civilian market exists at present for this vaccine.

IMPACT ON THE ARMED FORCES

Military surveillance data show minimal adenovirus-related morbidity during the period when the adenovirus vaccine was available and used at the training installations, followed by increased infection rates and hospitalization as vaccine administration became limited and finally ceased. Between October 1996 and May 1998, among symptomatic trainees at four sites, those who did not receive type 4 and 7 vaccine were 13 times more likely to have a positive adenovirus culture and 28 times more likely to be positive for type 4 or 7 adenovirus.[3] Ft. Jackson, Ft. Gordon, NTC Great Lakes, Cape May, Ft. Leonard Wood, Lackland AFB, and, most recently, Ft. Benning, have reported adenovirus epidemics, some with serious morbidity. Some epidemics have required adjustments such as the realignment of resources to convert barracks to infirmaries, the opening of new infirmary wards, the cancellation of elective surgeries, and staffing shifts. A few training camps have seen increases—20-fold at one base—in recruit recycling, when recruits miss enough of the training program that they need to begin again. The published surveillance data graphically show the temporal relationship between vaccine administration and respiratory disease rates in training camps.[4]

---

[1]Russell PK. Adenovirus infection is not trivial. *U.S. Medicine*, November 1998.

[2]Barraza EM, Ludwig SL, Gaydos JC, Brundage JF. Reemergence of adenovirus type 4 acute respiratory disease in military trainees: Report of an outbreak during a lapse in vaccination. *Journal of Infectious Diseases* 179, 1999.

[3]Gray GC, Goswani PR, Malasig MD, Hawksworth AW, Trump DH, Ryan MA, Schnurr DP (for the Adenovirus Surveillance Group). Adult adenovirus infections: Loss of orphaned vaccines precipitates military respiratory disease epidemics. *Clinical Infectious Diseases* 31:663-670, September 2000.

[4]Gray et al., *ibid.*

In the 1950s and 1960s, before military scientists identified the causative viruses and developed this effective and safe oral vaccine,[5,6,7] approximately 50 percent of recruits fell ill with acute respiratory disease, with certain sites reporting 80 percent attack rates in some years. The vaccine program cut those rates, and the associated hospitalizations, in half. A 1998 cost-effectiveness analysis, using incidence data, a range of vaccination policy options, and medical and training cost data, estimated a savings of approximately $16 million per year were the DoD to reinstate the vaccine program.[8]

CURRENT DEVELOPMENT EFFORT

Attempts by the DoD to find an alternative solution, including initial negotiations with another vaccine manufacturer, have been unsuccessful to date. To restart an adenovirus-vaccine program, the new manufacturer must go through the full FDA new-product approval process. With a one-time $14 million investment from the Defense Health Program, the Medical Research and Materiel Command is preparing a Request for Proposals (RFP). Challenges include creating a contract strategy, with elements such as commitments to multi-year funding, to which manufacturers might respond. DoD anticipates releasing the RFP for comments in the fall of 2000, working toward the best-and-final offer stage in January 2001. Even without schedule slippage, a vaccine will not be available for use within the next three years.[9] The initial funding amount likely will cover only Phase I preparation and some administrative and technical support.[10]

---

[5]Top FH Jr, Grossman RA, Bartelloni PJ, Segal HE, Dudding BA, Russell PK, Buescher EL. Immunization with live types 7 and 4 adenovirus vaccines. I. Safety, infectivity, antigenicity, and potency of adenovirus type 7 vaccine in humans. *Journal of Infectious Diseases* 124(2):148, August 1971.

[6]Rose HM, Lamson TH, Buescher EL. Adenoviral infection in military recruits: Emergence of type 7 and type 21 infections in recruits immunized with type 4 oral vaccine. *Arch Environ Health* 21:356, September 1970.

[7]Takafuji ET, Gaydos JC, Allen RG, Top FH Jr. Simultaneous administration of live, enteric-coated adenovirus types 4, 7, and 21 vaccines: Safety and immunogenicity. *Journal of Infectious Diseases* 140(1):48, July 1979.

[8]Howell MR, Nang RN, Gaydos CA, Gaydos JC. Prevention of adenoviral acute respiratory disease in Army recruits: Cost-effectiveness of a military vaccination policy. *American Journal of Preventive Medicine* 14(3), 1998.

[9]Howell W. Adenovirus history. Presentation to the Institute of Medicine Committee on a Strategy for Minimizing the Impact of Naturally Occurring Infectious Diseases of Military Importance: Vaccine Issues in the U.S. Military, September 2000.

[10]Howell W. Personal communication, October 2000.

DISCUSSION

- The DoD urgently needs adenovirus vaccine to (a) prevent increasingly large epidemics of febrile illness that put military personnel at risk of illness and even death,[11,12] and (b) avoid costs associated with medical care and disrupted or lost training days due to adenovirus illness.
- The military acquisition and procurement system has proven itself incapable of maintaining continuous availability of the adenovirus vaccine, and, in the opinion of the committee, its structure is inadequate to avoid similar failures for other limited use vaccine products.
- Although the commitment of $14 million of Defense Health Program funding is welcome, it is clearly not sufficient to reestablish licensure and ensure continued manufacture and purchase of an adenovirus vaccine. It seems unlikely that a commitment of this magnitude will be sufficient to bring competent, experienced manufacturers of vaccines into the negotiation process. The likelihood of restoring adenovirus vaccine to the military is significantly threatened by the lack of a longer range funding commitment.
- Reinstating the adenovirus vaccine program would be cost-effective. The monetary benefits of this vaccine's use unequivocably outweigh the high initial expenditures.

♦ ♦ ♦ ♦ ♦ ♦ ♦

Military service places young recruits in a uniquely high-risk setting for adenovirus infections during their training. Therefore, the Department of Defense has an obligation to protect recruits against this well-defined and largely preventable infection. To date, military training operations have not been perceived as significantly affected by adenovirus vaccine unavailability, as indicated by the relative lack of attention given the situation by upper-level commanders. However, the ongoing health surveillance, epidemiology, and military preventive medicine networks have gathered incontrovertible evidence of an impending public health emergency.

Sincerely,

Stanley M. Lemon, M.D. (*Chair*), for the Institute of Medicine
Committee on a Strategy for Minimizing the Impact of Naturally Occurring Infectious Diseases of Military Importance: Vaccine Issues in the U.S. Military

---

[11]Levin S, Dietrich J, Guillory J. Fatal nonbacterial pneumonia associated with Adenovirus type 4: Occurrence in an adult. *Journal of the American Medical Association* 201:975, 1967.

[12]Dudding B, Wagner S, Zeller J. Fatal pneumonia associated with adenovirus type 7 in three military trainees. *New England Journal of Medicine* 286:1289, 1972.

INSTITUTE OF MEDICINE • 2101 Constitution Avenue, N.W. • Washington, DC 20418

NOTICE: The project that is the subject of this report was approved by the Governing Board of the National Research Council, whose members are drawn from the councils of the National Academy of Sciences, the National Academy of Engineering, and the Institute of Medicine. The members of the committee responsible for the report were chosen for their special competences and with regard for appropriate balance.

Support for this project was provided by the U.S. Army Medical Research and Materiel Command under Contract No. DAMD17-00-C-0003. The views, opinions, and/or findings contained in this report are those of the Institute of Medicine Committee on a Strategy for Minimizing the Impact of Naturally Occurring Infectious Diseases of Military Importance: Vaccine Issues in the U.S. Military and should not be construed as an official Department of the Army position, policy, or decision unless so designated by other documentation.

Additional copies of this report are available in limited quantities from the Medical Follow-up Agency, 2101 Constitution Avenue, N.W., Washington, DC 20418. The full text of this report is available on line at **www.nap.edu.**

For more information about the Institute of Medicine, visit the IOM home page at **www.iom.edu.**

Copyright 2000 by the National Academy of Sciences. All rights reserved.

Printed in the United States of America.

"Knowing is not enough; we must apply.
Willing is not enough; we must do."
—Goethe

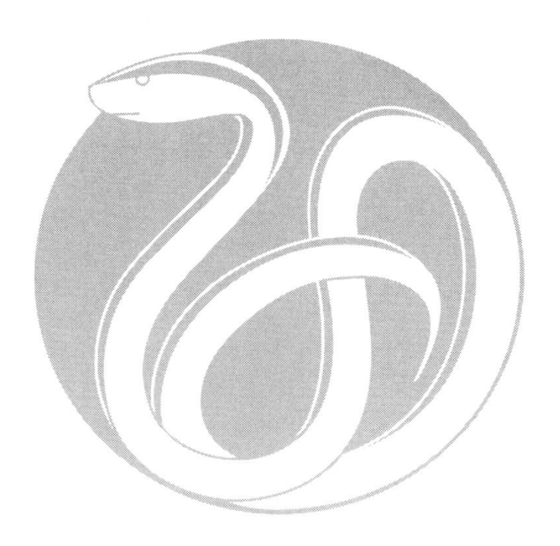

INSTITUTE OF MEDICINE

Shaping the Future for Health

THE NATIONAL ACADEMIES

National Academy of Sciences
National Academy of Engineering
Institute of Medicine
National Research Council

The **National Academy of Sciences** is a private, nonprofit, self-perpetuating society of distinguished scholars engaged in scientific and engineering research, dedicated to the furtherance of science and technology and to their use for the general welfare. Upon the authority of the charter granted to it by the Congress in 1863, the Academy has a mandate that requires it to advise the federal government on scientific and technical matters. Dr. Bruce M. Alberts is president of the National Academy of Sciences.

The **National Academy of Engineering** was established in 1964, under the charter of the National Academy of Sciences, as a parallel organization of outstanding engineers. It is autonomous in its administration and in the selection of its members, sharing with the National Academy of Sciences the responsibility for advising the federal government. The National Academy of Engineering also sponsors engineering programs aimed at meeting national needs, encourages education and research, and recognizes the superior achievements of engineers. Dr. William A. Wulf is president of the National Academy of Engineering.

The **Institute of Medicine** was established in 1970 by the National Academy of Sciences to secure the services of eminent members of appropriate professions in the examination of policy matters pertaining to the health of the public. The Institute acts under the responsibility given to the National Academy of Sciences by its congressional charter to be an adviser to the federal government and, upon its own initiative, to identify issues of medical care, research, and education. Dr. Kenneth I. Shine is president of the Institute of Medicine.

The **National Research Council** was organized by the National Academy of Sciences in 1916 to associate the broad community of science and technology with the Academy's purposes of furthering knowledge and advising the federal government. Functioning in accordance with general policies determined by the Academy, the Council has become the principal operating agency of both the National Academy of Sciences and the National Academy of Engineering in providing services to the government, the public, and the scientific and engineering communities. The Council is administered jointly by both Academies and the Institute of Medicine. Dr. Bruce M. Alberts and Dr. William A. Wulf are chairman and vice chairman, respectively, of the National Research Council.

COMMITTEE ON A STRATEGY FOR MINIMIZING THE IMPACT OF NATURALLY OCCURRING INFECTIOUS DISEASES OF MILITARY IMPORTANCE: VACCINE ISSUES IN THE U.S. MILITARY

Stanley M. Lemon, M.D. (*Chair*), Dean of Medicine and Professor, University of Texas Medical Branch, Galveston
Charles C. J. Carpenter, M.D., Professor of Medicine, Brown University, The Miriam Hospital, Providence, Rhode Island
Ciro A. de Quadros, M.D., M.P.H., Director, Division of Vaccines and Immunization, Pan American Health Organization, Washington, D.C.
R. Gordon Douglas, Jr., M.D., Princeton, New Jersey
Lawrence O. Gostin, J.D., LL.D. (Hon.), Co-Director, Georgetown/Johns Hopkins Joint Program in Public Health and Law, and Professor of Law, Georgetown University
M. Carolyn Hardegree, M.D., Potomac, Maryland
Samuel L. Katz, M.D., Wilburt C. Davison Professor and Chairman Emeritus, Duke University Medical Center
F. Marc LaForce, M.D., BASICS II, Arlington, Virginia
Stanley A. Plotkin, M.D., Doylestown, Pennsylvania
Gregory A. Poland, M.D., Chief, Mayo Vaccine Research Group, Mayo Clinic and Foundation, Rochester, Minnesota
N. Regina Rabinovich, M.D., M.P.H., Director, Malaria Vaccine Initiative, Program for Appropriate Technology in Health, Rockville, Maryland
Philip K. Russell, M.D., Potomac, Maryland
Ronald J. Saldarini, Ph.D., Mahwah, New Jersey
Mary E. Wilson, M.D., Chief of Infectious Diseases, Mount Auburn Hospital, Cambridge, Massachusetts, Associate Professor of Medicine, Harvard Medical School

Staff

Susan Thaul, Ph.D., Study Director
Karen Kazmerzak, Research Assistant
Richard N. Miller, M.D., M.P.H., Director, Medical Follow-up Agency
Heather O'Maonaigh, M.A., Program Officer
Pamela Ramey-McCray, Administrative Assistant

INDEPENDENT REPORT REVIEWERS

This report has been reviewed in draft form by individuals chosen for their diverse perspectives and technical expertise, in accordance with procedures approved by the NRC's Report Review Committee. The purpose of this independent review is to provide candid and critical comments that will assist the institution in making its published report as sound as possible and to ensure that the report meets institutional standards for objectivity, evidence, and responsiveness to the study charge. The review comments and draft manuscript remain confidential to protect the integrity of the deliberative process. We wish to thank the following individuals for their review of this report:

Robert B. Couch, M.D., Baylor College of Medicine
Bernard Gert, Ph.D., Dartmouth College
James W. LeDuc, Ph.D., Centers for Disease Control and Prevention
Adel A.F. Mahmoud, M.D., Ph.D., Merck & Co., Inc.
Bernhard T. Mittemeyer, M.D., Surgeon General, US Army, ret., Texas Tech University
William Schaffner, M.D., Vanderbilt University

Although the reviewers listed above have provided many constructive comments and suggestions, they were not asked to endorse the conclusions or recommendations nor did they see the final draft of the report before its release. The review of this report was overseen by D.A. Henderson M.D., M.P.H. of The Johns Hopkins University, appointed jointly by the Institute of Medicine and the NRC's Report Review Committee, who was responsible for making certain that an independent examination of this report was carried out in accordance with institutional procedures and that all review comments were carefully considered. Responsibility for the final content of this report rests entirely with the authoring committee and the institution.

Appendix B

Open Meeting Agendas

Meeting I
April 3 and 4, 2000
The Foundry Building, Washington, D.C.

3 April 2000

10:00AM Sponsor Presentation: Charge to the IOM and Welcoming Remarks
MG John S. Parker, M.D.,
Commanding General
U.S. Army Medical Research and Materiel Command

Overview of the Military Infectious Diseases Research Program
COL Charles H. Hoke, Jr., M.D.,
Research Area Director
Military Infectious Diseases Research Program

11:00AM Break

11:15AM Sponsor Presentation, continued
Overview of the DoD Research and Development (Acquisition) Model
COL Rodney A. Michael, M.D.
Research Area Deputy Director
Military Infectious Diseases Research Program

Biologic Warfare Defense Research and Endemic Infectious Diseases Research: Whence and why the dichotomy
COL John F. Glenn, Ph.D.
Deputy for Research and Development
U.S. Army Medical Research and Materiel Command

12:15PM Lunch

1:15PM Discussion with Sponsor:
Current challenges
Overview of the challenges to adequate vaccine strategy presented by industry and DoD policies and constraints
Overview of the regulatory parameters that currently affect military vaccine strategy
Discussion of what the U.S. Army seeks to gain from this committee report
Discussion of charge

2:15PM Break, end of open session

Meeting II
June 19 and 20, 2000
The Foundry Building, Washington, D.C.

19 June 2000

10:00AM Welcome and Introduction
Stanley Lemon, M.D., Chair

10:05AM Examples of the Impact of Vaccine Preventable Infectious Disease:

Impact of Recent Adenovirus Outbreaks in Military Training Centers
CAPT Gregory Gray, M.D., M.P.H.
Director, DoD Center for Deployment Health Research
Naval Health Research Center, San Diego

Lt Col James Neville, M.D., M.P.H.
Chief, Force Health Protection and Surveillance Branch
U.S. Air Force Institute for Environment, Safety & Occupational Health Risk Analysis
Brooks Air Force Base

Leonard N. Binn, Ph.D.
Supervisory Research Microbiologist, Department of Virus Diseases
Walter Reed Army Institute of Research

The Meningococcal Meningitis Situation, Military and Civilian
Juliette Morgan, M.D.
Medical Epidemiologist, Meningitis and Special Pathogens Branch
Centers for Disease Control and Prevention

John Brundage, M.D., M.P.H.
Senior Research Epidemiologist, Henry M. Jackson Foundation
Army Medical Surveillance Activity
Walter Reed Army Institute of Research

11:30AM JVAP—Procurement Process for Vaccines for Biowarfare Defense
Richard B. Paul, M.A.
Acting Program Manager, Joint Vaccine Acquisition Program

12:00PM Vaccine Development Success–Policy Failure
Adenovirus Vaccine: Successful Development
Franklin H. Top, Jr., M.D.
Executive Vice President and Medical Director,
MedImmune

Adenovirus Vaccine: A Policy Failure
Joel Gaydos, M.D., M.P.H.
DoD Global Emerging Infections Surveillance & Response System,
Division of Preventive Medicine, Walter Reed Army Institute of
Research

12:45PM Lunch (and continued discussion)

1:30PM Vaccine Research & Development: Priority Setting
DoD Requirements Generation and Acquisition
James H. Nelson, Ph.D.
Director, U.S. Army Medical Materiel Development Activity

Military Medical Surveillance of Infectious Disease
LTC Mark V. Rubertone, M.D., M.P.H.
Chief, Army Medical Surveillance Activity
U.S. Army Center for Health Promotion and Preventive Medicine

Medical Intelligence
Deborah G. Keimig, Ph.D.
Chief, Epidemiology and Environmental Health Division
Armed Forces Medical Intelligence Center, Fort Detrick

Priority Setting in Practice
COL Rodney A. Michael, M.D.
Deputy Director, Military Infectious Disease Research Program

Discussion

4:00PM Open session ends

20 June 2000

7:30AM Continental Breakfast

8:00AM Review of Meeting Day 1 and Introduction of Day 2 Program
Stanley Lemon, M.D., Chair

8:20AM Status of Limited Use Vaccines in the Military
LTC Phillip R. Pittman, M.D., M.P.H.
Senior Medical Scientist
U.S. Army Research Institute of Infectious Diseases

8:50AM How Others (Try to) Make Limited Use Vaccine Development Work:

Food and Drug Administration
Karen Goldenthal, M.D.
Director, Division of Vaccines & Related Products Applications

National Institute of Allergy and Infectious Disease, National Institutes of Health
Carole A. Heilman, Ph.D.
Director, Division of Microbiology and Infectious Diseases

Centers for Disease Control and Prevention
James W. LeDuc, Ph.D.
Acting Director, Division of Viral and Rickettsial Diseases
National Center for Infectious Diseases
Centers for Disease Control and Prevention

Industry Involvement in Federal Vaccine Development and Procurement Efforts
Thomas P. Monath, M.D.
Vice President, Research & Medical Affairs, OraVax Inc.

Discussion: Constraints Faced and Handled
How Might DoD Use These Approaches

11:45AM Lunch—with concurrent discussion based on morning's presentations
Open session ends

Meeting III
September 21 and 22, 2000
The Foundry Building, Washington, D.C.

21 September 2000

11:00AM Welcome
Stanley Lemon, M.D., Chair

11:05AM Adenovirus vaccine
MAJ Michael Dyer, M.S.
Office of the TRADOC Surgeon
William Howell
Deputy for Acquisition and Advanced Development
U.S. Army Medical Research and Materiel Command

12:00PM Lunch

12:45PM Vaccine production
Gary Nabel, M.D., Ph.D.
Director, NIH Vaccine Research Center
Jack Melling, Ph.D.
formerly with the Salk Institute and the Center for Applied Microbiology and Research

2:00PM Priorities
LTC Brian G. Scott, M.D.
Clinical Consultant, Force Protection AMEDD Center and School
Directorate of Combat and Doctrine Development

COL John Frazier Glenn, Ph.D.
Deputy for Research and Development
U.S. Army Medical Research and Materiel Command

Discussion
Presenters along with:
COL Charles Hoke, Jr., M.D.
COL Rodney Michael, M.D.

4:00PM Discussion
5:00PM Adjourn for the day

Meeting IV
November 13 and 14, 2000
The Foundry Building, Washington, D.C.

13 November 2000

9:30AM Continental breakfast in conference room

10:00AM Review agenda, introduce speakers

10:10AM Incentivizing limited use vaccine production: getting and keeping vaccines
Kevin L. Reilly
President, Wyeth Vaccines, Wyeth Pharmaceuticals

11:30AM Public release of this committee's interim report:
Urgent Attention Needed to Restore Lapsed Adenovirus Vaccine Availability: A Letter Report
Stanley Lemon, M.D., Chair

Adenovirus update
CDR Jeff Yund, M.D.
Division of Preventive Medicine and Occupational Health
U.S. Navy Bureau of Medicine and Surgery

12:30PM Working lunch in conference room for committee, staff, and guests

1:30PM Priority setting revisited (panel discussion)
COL John Frazier Glenn, Ph.D.
Deputy for Research and Development
U.S. Army Medical Research and Materiel Command

LTC Brian G. Scott, M.D.
Clinical Consultant, Force Protection
Directorate of Combat and Doctrine Development
AMEDD Center & School

COL Charles Hoke, Jr., M.D.
Director, Military Infectious Diseases Research Program
U.S. Army Medical Research and Materiel Command

3:00PM Open session ends

Meeting V
Tuesday, February 27, 2001
The Foundry Building, Washington, D.C.

12:00PM Working lunch in conference room for committee, staff, and guests

1:00PM Setting vaccine priorities in DoD
Anna Johnson-Winegar, Ph.D.
Deputy Assistant to the Secretary of Defense
Counterproliferation and Chemical/Biological Defense

2:00PM Open session ends

Appendix C

Committee and Staff Biographies

COMMITTEE MEMBERS

STANLEY M. LEMON, M.D. (Chair), is dean of the School of Medicine, University of Texas Medical Branch at Galveston, in addition to his current service as professor of microbiology and immunology and internal medicine. A graduate of Princeton University and the University of Rochester School of Medicine and Dentistry, he has previously held academic appointments at the University of North Carolina at Chapel Hill and served from 1977 to 1983 as a staff physician and as an infectious disease officer at the Walter Reed Army Institute of Research. He serves as chair of the U.S. Hepatitis Panel of the U.S.–Japan Cooperative Medical Science Program (U.S. Public Health Service) and as vice chair of the Forum on Emerging Infections of the Board on Global Health (Institute of Medicine). He has previously chaired the Advisory Committee on Vaccines and Related Biologics of the Center for Biologics Evaluation and Research (Food and Drug Administration) and the Steering Committee on Poliovirus and Hepatitis Viruses of the Programme for Vaccine Development (World Health Organization). He has served on the Executive Committee of the International Committee on the Taxonomy of Viruses (International Union of Microbiologic Sciences) and the Nominating Committee of the American Society for the Advancement of Science. His professional society memberships include the American Clinical and Climatologic Society, the Association of American Physicians, the American Society for Clinical Investigation, the Infectious Diseases Society of America, the American Society of Virology, and the American Society for Microbiology. Dr. Lemon is the recipient of the Meritorious Service Medal, U.S. Army (1983), and the Commissioner's Special Citation, Food and Drug Administration (1996).

CHARLES C. J. CARPENTER, M.D., is professor of medicine at Brown University and director of the Brown University International Health Institute. He is a member of the Institute of Medicine and has held offices in several national professional organizations. He chairs the AIDS Research Advisory Committee of the National Institutes of Health, is a member of the Committee on Guidelines for Antiretroviral Therapy of the Department of Health and Human Services, was a member of the Institute of Medicine panel on Priorities in Vaccine Development, and has served on numerous scientific advisory committees and panels. He is a principal investigator associated with the Lifespan/Tufts/Brown Center for AIDS Research, is the chair of the U.S. Delegation of the U.S.–Japan Cooperative Medical Sciences Program, and has served as chair of the American Board of Internal Medicine and as president of the Association of American Physicians. He has received several awards for outstanding contributions to medicine.

CIRO A. de QUADROS, M.D., M.P.H., is director of the Division of Vaccines and Immunization, Pan American Health Organization. Dr. de Quadros served as a member of the Institute of Medicine Committee on Microbial Threats to Health and as a member of the Institute of Medicine Steering Committee on the Children's Vaccine Initiative. He is a member of the American Public Health Association, the American Association for the Advancement of Science, the Global Health Council, the American Society for Tropical Medicine and Hygiene, and the European Society of Microbiology and Infectious Disease. His areas of interest and expertise include epidemiology, disease control, maternal and child health, vaccinology, and vaccine research. Dr. de Quadros has received many honors and awards including the 1988 Dean's Medal awarded by the Johns Hopkins University School of Hygiene and Public Health, the 1990 International Child Survival Award from the USA Committee for UNICEF and the Carter Center, and the year 2000 Albert B. Sabin Gold Medal awarded by the Sabin Vaccine Institute.

R. GORDON DOUGLAS, Jr., M.D., is a former president of the Merck Vaccine Division, Merck & Co. Inc., (he retired in May 1999). Until his retirement, he was primarily responsible for the research, development, and manufacturing and marketing of Merck's vaccine products. Prior to joining Merck in 1989, Dr. Douglas was a career physician and academician, specializing in infectious diseases. From 1982 to 1990 he was professor of medicine and chairman, Department of Medicine, Cornell University Medical College, and physician-in-chief, The New York Hospital. He also served as head of the Infectious Disease Unit at the University of Rochester School of Medicine. Dr. Douglas is a graduate of Princeton University and Cornell University Medical College. He is a member of the Institute of Medicine, the Association of American Physicians, the Infectious Diseases Society of America, and numerous other organizations and has served on the National Vaccine Advisory Committee.

LAWRENCE O. GOSTIN, J.D., LL.D. (Hon.), is professor of law at Georgetown University Law Center, professor of law and public health at the Johns Hopkins University School of Hygiene and Public Health, and co-director of the Johns Hopkins/Georgetown Program on Law and Public Health. Professor Gostin is a visiting scholar at the Centre for Socio-Legal Studies, Oxford University. He is also a fellow of the Kennedy Institute of Ethics of Georgetown University and a member of the Steering and Executive Committees of the Georgetown University Institute for Health Care Research and Policy. Professor Gostin is the editor of the "Health Law and Ethics" section of the *Journal of the American Medical Association*. Professor Gostin has served as a member of many Institute of Medicine committees, including the Committee on Battlefield Radiation Exposure Criteria. He is a member of the Institute of Medicine Board on Health Promotion and Disease Prevention.

M. CAROLYN HARDEGREE, M.D., recently retired as director of the Office of Vaccines Research and Review, Center for Biologics Evaluation and Research, Food and Drug Administration. She serves as a member of the World Health Organization Steering Committee on Immunization Safety and as a member of the National Vaccine Advisory Committee's Pandemic Influenza Working Group. She has previously served as a member or liaison of various government and nongovernment committees and groups, including the Institute of Medicine Vaccine Safety Forum and the Institute of Medicine Committee to Study the Interaction of Drugs, Biologics, and Chemicals in Deployed U.S. Military Forces. Dr. Hardegree's research has been in the area of bacterial toxins and vaccines. Her honors include the Department of Health and Human Services Secretary's Award for Distinguished Service and the Food and Drug Administration Distinguished Alumnus Award.

SAMUEL L. KATZ, M.D., is the Wilburt Cornell Davison Professor and chairman emeritus of pediatrics at Duke University. His career has been devoted to infectious disease research, focusing principally on vaccine research and development. Dr. Katz's research included an extensive collaborative effort with Nobel Laureate John F. Enders at Boston Children's Hospital, during which time they developed the attenuated measles virus vaccine now used throughout the world. Dr. Katz has chaired the Committee on Infectious Diseases of the American Academy of Pediatrics (the Redbook Committee), the Advisory Committee on Immunization Practices of the Centers for Disease Control and Prevention, several World Health Organization panels and panels on the Children's Vaccine Initiative and human immunodeficiency virus. He has been president of the American Pediatric Society and the Association of Medical School Pediatric Department chair. He is the coeditor (with A. Gershon and P. Hotez) of a textbook (now in its tenth edition) on infectious diseases. He chaired the Board of the

Burroughs Wellcome Fund. Dr. Katz is a member of the Institute of Medicine and has been a member of many Institute of Medicine committees including the Committee on Establishing Vaccine Development Priorities for the United States (1995–1999), the Forum on Emerging Infections (1996–1999), the Committee on Child Health in the Former Yugoslavia (1995), the Committee for the Children's Vaccine Initiative—Continuing Activities (1995), the Committee for a Study of Public/Private Sector Relations in Vaccine Innovation (1985), and the Committee on Issues and Priorities for New Vaccine Development (1982–1986).

F. MARC LaFORCE, M.D., has recently become the director of the Meningitis Vaccine Project, a joint endeavor between the World Health Organization and the Program for Appropriate Technology in Health. Dr. LaForce has had a long-standing interest in national and international immunization policies. He has held academic appointments at the University of Colorado and the University of Rochester, where he is now a clinical professor of medicine. Dr. LaForce has also served as the director of BASICS II, a large child survival project funded by the U.S. Agency for International Development, and as an epidemic intelligence service officer in the U.S. Public Health Service. He is a member of the American Epidemiological Society, the Society of General Internal Medicine, and the Society of Hospital Epidemiologists of America.

STANLEY A. PLOTKIN, M.D., is a medical and scientific consultant, Aventis Pasteur, after 7 years as medical and scientific director, Pasteur Merieux Connaught Vaccines, Paris, France. He is also emeritus professor of pediatrics at the University of Pennsylvania and emeritus professor of virology at the Wistar Institute. Over the course of his career he has served as senior assistant surgeon, Epidemic Intelligence Service, U.S. Public Health Service, and as associate chairman, Department of Pediatrics, University of Pennsylvania. Dr. Plotkin has developed many vaccines, including the rubella vaccine, RA27/3 strain, now exclusively used in the United States and throughout the world. He has held editorial positions with many scholarly journals and is a member of numerous professional and scientific societies, including the American Association for the Advancement of Science, the Society for Pediatric Research, the American Society for Microbiology, the Infectious Diseases Society of America, and the American Epidemiologic Society. Dr. Plotkin has received several professional awards including the French Legion Medal of Honor (1998); the Clinical Virology Award, Pan American Group for Rapid Viral Diagnosis (1995); the Distinguished Physician Award, Pediatric Infectious Disease Society (1993); and the Bruce Medal of the American College of Physicians (1987).

GREGORY A. POLAND, M.D., is professor of medicine, infectious diseases, molecular pharmacology, and experimental therapeutics, Mayo Medical School. He is vice chair of the Department of Medicine for Research and director of the

Mayo Vaccine Group. He is president of the International Society for Vaccines and American editor for the journal *Vaccine*. He also directs the Outpatient General Clinical Research Center and Immunization Clinic and Services for the Mayo Clinic. His professional memberships include the International Society for Vaccines, the National Coalition for Adult Immunization, the Infectious Diseases Society of America, and the American College of Physicians. He also serves as a member of the U.S. Department of Health and Human Services' Healthy People 2010 Immunization and Infectious Diseases Objectives Working Group, the National Vaccine Advisory Committee, and the U.S. Public Health Service Advisory Committee on Immunization Practice: Vaccination and Bioterrorism.

N. REGINA RABINOVICH, M.D., M.P.H., is director of the Malaria Health Initiative, which is funded by a grant from the Bill and Melinda Gates Foundation, administered by the Program for Appropriate Technology in Health. Previously, she served as the chief of the Clinical and Regulatory Affairs Branch and the Clinical Studies Section of the Division of Microbiology and Infectious Diseases, National Institute of Allergy and Infectious Diseases, National Institutes of Health. Dr. Rabinovich serves as a consultant for the Vaccines and Related Biologicals Advisory Committee, Food and Drug Administration. In the past she has served as National Institutes of Health liaison to the Centers for Disease Control and Prevention Committee on Immunization Practices and as chair of the Epidemiology Section of the American Academy of Pediatrics.

PHILIP K. RUSSELL, M.D., recently became a special advisor on vaccine development and production to the newly created Office of Public Health Preparedness, Department of Health and Human Services. Dr. Russell is also professor emeritus, Department of International Health, at the Johns Hopkins University School of Hygiene and Public Health. From 1959 to 1990 he served in the U.S. Army Medical Corps, retiring as a Major General and Assistant Surgeon General for Research and Development. He has expertise in infectious diseases, tropical medicine, virology, immunology, and vaccines. Dr. Russell has served on the Board of Scientific Counselors for the Centers for Disease Control and Prevention's Center for Infectious Diseases, the Scientific Advisory Group of Experts for the World Health Organization Programme on Vaccine Development, the Presidential Advisory Committee on Human Radiation Experiments, Defense Science Board task forces on chemical weapons and biological defense, and numerous committees of the National Academies. He has received the Order of Military Medical Merit and the Distinguished Service Medal and is a fellow of the American Academy of Microbiology and the Infectious Diseases Society of America.

RONALD J. SALDARINI, Ph.D., retired in 1999 as president of Wyeth-Lederle Vaccines & Pediatrics business group. Before joining American Home Products

Corporation, Dr. Saldarini was president of the Lederle Praxis Biologicals Division of the American Cyanamid Company. He is on the Board of Trustees of the National Foundation of Infectious Diseases and the Infectious Disease Institute of New Jersey. He is a member of the Board of Directors Partnership for Prevention, the Presidents Corporate Council for the Children's Health Fund, the Board of Directors of the Institute for the Advanced Studies of Immunology and Aging, the Policy Board of the Albert B. Sabin Vaccine Foundation, and the Immunization Advisory Council of the New York State Department of Health. He remains a member of several professional societies including Sigma Xi.

MARY E. WILSON, M.D., is associate professor of medicine, Harvard Medical School; associate professor, Department of Population and International Health, Harvard School of Public Health; and chief of infectious diseases, Mount Auburn Hospital. She is also the author and editor of numerous books and articles including *Disease in Evolution: Global Changes and Emergence of Infectious Disease.* Dr. Wilson serves as a consultant on the Travel Advisory Board of Merck & Co.'s Vaccine Division. She is a member of the editorial advisory boards of the journals *Global Change and Human Health*, *Clinical Infectious Diseases*, and *Emerging Infectious Diseases*. Dr. Wilson has served on the Institute of Medicine Committee on the Elimination of Tuberculosis in the United States and the Advisory Committee on Immunization Practices of the Centers for Disease Control and Prevention and currently serves on the Institute of Medicine Committee on Microbial Threats to Health in the 21st Century.

STUDY STAFF

SUSAN THAUL, Ph.D., is the director of this study. With the Medical Follow-up Agency of the Institute of Medicine, she produced *The Five Series Study: Mortality of Military Participants in U.S. Nuclear Weapons Tests* (2000) and the 1999 report *Potential Radiation Exposure in Military Operations: Protecting the Soldier Before, During, and After* and coauthored the 1996 report *Mortality of Veteran Participants in the CROSSROADS Nuclear Test.* Dr. Thaul had previously led Institute of Medicine projects in women's health, national statistics, and health services research, among others. She received a Ph.D. in epidemiology from Columbia University and an M.S. in health policy and management from Harvard University. Heading the health staff of the U.S. Senate Committee on Veterans' Affairs (then chaired by Senator Alan Cranston), Dr. Thaul developed legislation in preventive health care and research, women's health care, sexual assault services and prevention, nurse and physician pay, and health effects of environmental hazards during service. Earlier positions were with the Agency for Healthcare Research and Quality, the Harlem Hospital Prevention of Prematurity Project, and the New York City Health and Hospitals Corporation.

SALEM FISSEHA is a research assistant with the Medical Follow-up Agency, Institute of Medicine. She received a bachelor of arts degree in anthropology from Harvard College in 1997. She plans to pursue a master's degree at the London School of Hygiene and Tropical Medicine in September 2002.

RICHARD N. MILLER, M.D., M.P.H., is the director of the Medical Follow-up Agency of the Institute of Medicine, a position he took upon retiring, as Colonel, from the U.S. Army. Dr. Miller's work in infectious diseases research, teaching of the Army Tropical Medicine Course, and serving as the Director of the Preventive Medicine Residency at Walter Reed Army Institute of Research capped a career of almost thirty years in military preventive medicine and public health, a large part of which was spent in overseas locations.

HEATHER O'MAONAIGH, M.A., has served as a staff member with the Institute of Medicine since 1998. She holds a master's degree in demography from Georgetown University and a bachelor of science degree in sociology from Western Washington University.

PAMELA RAMEY-McCRAY is the administrative assistant for the Medical Follow-up Agency.